Obstacle Race Training Bible

James Villepigue, CSCS

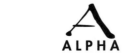

ALPHA
A member of Penguin Group (USA) Inc.

ALPHA BOOKS

Published by Penguin Group (USA) Inc.

Penguin Group (USA) Inc., 375 Hudson Street, New York, New York 10014, USA • Penguin Group (Canada), 90 Eglinton Avenue East, Suite 700, Toronto, Ontario M4P 2Y3, Canada (a division of Pearson Penguin Canada Inc.) • Penguin Books Ltd., 80 Strand, London WC2R 0RL, England • Penguin Ireland, 25 St. Stephen's Green, Dublin 2, Ireland (a division of Penguin Books Ltd.) • Penguin Group (Australia), 250 Camberwell Road, Camberwell, Victoria 3124, Australia (a division of Pearson Australia Group Pty. Ltd.) • Penguin Books India Pvt. Ltd., 11 Community Centre, Panchsheel Park, New Delhi—110 017, India • Penguin Group (NZ), 67 Apollo Drive, Rosedale, North Shore, Auckland 1311, New Zealand (a division of Pearson New Zealand Ltd.) • Penguin Books (South Africa) (Pty.) Ltd., 24 Sturdee Avenue, Rosebank, Johannesburg 2196, South Africa • Penguin Books Ltd., Registered Offices: 80 Strand, London WC2R 0RL, England

International Standard Book Number: 978-1-61564-205-2
Library of Congress Catalog Card Number: 2012941770

14   13   12   8   7   6   5   4   3   2   1

Interpretation of the printing code: The rightmost number of the first series of numbers is the year of the book's printing; the rightmost number of the second series of numbers is the number of the book's printing. For example, a printing code of 12-1 shows that the first printing occurred in 2012.

Printed in the United States of America

Contents

Introduction

Like a spark hitting a drought-stricken forest floor on a breezy day, obstacle races and similar challenges have taken off like wildfire. A clever combination of trail races, military-style obstacle courses, mud runs, and backcountry adventures, obstacle races have captured the imagination of millions of people—athletes and nonathletes alike—who seek new thrills and challenges. A quick internet search turns up hundreds of obstacle races, many of them small, local events. Several races have literally taken to the road, hosting challenges around the United States and Canada, as well as England and Europe. They've developed large fan bases and have thousands of followers on Facebook. These social media outlets fan the flames of interest by allowing participants to post pictures and videos of themselves conquering the obstacles and whooping it up at the postrace parties these events are known for. They also provide a forum for sharing training tips and strategies for overcoming obstacles.

Because of their unique nature, obstacle races pose a training challenge. If you simply adopt a road racing training program, you'll be unprepared for the obstacles and other challenges these events throw your way. A straightforward bodybuilding program fails to take into account both the cardiovascular endurance required for the running component, and the functional skills involved in tackling the obstacles and challenges. And while many of the events featured in this book claim on their websites that very little training is required, that's a recipe for failure or even injury. What's the point of paying good money to enter an obstacle race if you have to skip most of the obstacles because you're too weak, tired, and out-of-shape to do them? Or even worse, you miss out because you pull a muscle a third of the way into the course.

That's where the *Obstacle Race Training Bible* comes in. In this book, I not only provide you with an eight-week training program for conquering any course, I also offer expert strategies and specific exercises for tackling 30 of the most common obstacles. And the beauty of my program is that it's not a one-size-fits-all endeavor. After taking a quick fitness assessment, you will know whether you should adopt the beginner, intermediate, or advanced training program, which are outlined in Chapter 11. Each program considers your base strengths and weaknesses, and builds from there.

Before setting out on a training program, you need to decide on an obstacle race that matches up with your goals. Some races appeal to hardcore competitors, while others draw weekend warriors. I provide an overview of 15 popular obstacle events in Chapter 2. While the races highlighted in Chapter 2 by no means comprise an exhaustive list—there are hundreds of local races, with new ones popping up all the time—the obstacles and other military-style challenges featured do cover the spectrum of events in the obstacle racing genre. Gateway races, such as the Warrior Dash and Superhero Scramble, are ideal for beginners; moderately difficult events, such as Tough Mudder, Spartan Sprint, and Rugged Maniac, are more appropriate for people who have put in some training time; and more hardcore events, such as the Super Spartan and Spartan Beast, are reserved for the most serious athletes.

When it's all said and done, participating in an obstacle race is all about challenging yourself while having the time of your life. You'll have a lot more fun during the race if you prepare in advance by choosing a race wisely, plan your strategy for attacking the obstacles, and train like the well-conditioned athlete that you already are, or have always wanted to be.

Acknowledgments

I am truly honored to dedicate this work of art to the most important people in my life.

To my beautiful wife, Heather, thank you for being my rock and for standing close by my side these last nine years. My life would not be as incredible as it is without you, baby … I love you!

To my beautiful children, Sienna James, Kaiya Reece, and Colton James, I thank God for you every day! You are my heart and I am the luckiest dad in the world!

To my mom, Nancy, an authentic angel on Earth and the glue that has always kept my family together. I love you more than you could ever know!

To my very talented sister, Deborah. Always have, Always will, Debbie. I'm proud of you and I adore you!

Keeping his spirit alive, I'd like to honor my beloved father and best friend, James R. Villepigue. I am blessed to have had the opportunity to spend 32 years of my amazing life with you, my best pal and navigator. I miss you.

To all of my family, friends, and loyal fanbase, what else can I say other than I am grateful to you all!

To my heavenly Father above, Jesus Christ, I thank you for the biggest blessing in my life … You! Thank you for filling my life with love, happiness, and health. Amen.

I would like to thank the following people: my publisher, Mike Sanders; my editor, Jennifer Moore; my literary agent, Bob DeForeo; my dear friend, former Navy SEAL Lieutenant Stew Smith (SpecialOpsCombine.com); my good friend and second pair of eyes, Eric Su; my good friends, Joe Volgey and Rich Gaspari at Gaspari Nutrition; the two people who gave me my first shots at success: the late Robert Kennedy and Andrew Flach; the greatest obstacle racer today and my business partner, Hobie Call; Jeff Oconnel and the crew over at Bodybuilding.com; and finally, all of the amazing obstacle race owners and race organizers who I've had the pleasure of working with. Thanks to you all!

I believe Obstacle Racing can become a professional sport, and I am looking forward to being a part of the process for making that so. If you want to be a part of it, too, join the Conquer Any Course Community at facebook.com/conqueranycourse.

Great things to come!

Chapter 1

Beyond the Mud: The Obstacle Racing Phenomenon

More than 1 million people signed up for an obstacle race last year—and that number is expected to grow by leaps and bounds. The seven-figure milestone is particularly impressive considering how new the racing genre is. Muddy Buddy is the granddaddy on a national scale, dating back to 1999. Most of the others entered the foray much more recently. Warrior Dash, a favorite for novice racers, launched its first races in 2009. Tough Mudder and Spartan followed close on Warrior's heels, introducing their inaugural races in 2010.

What's behind this dramatic rise of interest in obstacle racing? And is it just a passing fad, or is the genre here to stay?

What's the Buzz All About?

Clearly, obstacle races meet a pent-up demand for new experiences and challenges. For many people, they provide a stiff dose of adventure without requiring distant travel or vast sums of money.

To better understand the attraction of obstacle races, it helps to consider what prompted their founders to start them in the first place. Tough Mudder, for example, was launched by Will Dean, a former British counterterrorism agent. While getting his MBA at Harvard, Dean was inspired to start Tough Mudder out of frustration with unimaginative and repetitive marathons, triathlons, mud runs, and other adventure runs. Spartan Race looked at the idea of military-style boot camps and wondered how to bring that level of challenge to weekend warriors and desk jockeys.

Note

Military units dating back to the ancient Greeks and Romans trained with rope courses. The Japanese military used obstacle courses starting around the 1800s. During World War II, Brigadier General William Hoge created an obstacle course of barbed wire, hurdles, ditches, pipes, and other challenges to train U.S. Army soldiers at Fort Belvoir in Virginia during World War II. After that course proved its effectiveness, the obstacle course was adopted at army installations throughout the country.

"In a marathon, I can tell you what the outcome is going to be. You know what you're in for. As opposed to these races—you never know what you're going to be faced with until you're there and you're doing it. That's so cool," said Carrie Adams, brand manager for Spartan Races and a long-time competitor. "It really appeals to me because you kinda get bored in your day-to-day racing."

The grueling nature of the obstacles interjects an element of wildness into a routine life. Adams said, "People are looking for ways to get back to the primal roots that we've all gotten disconnected from. You go back to work on Monday and are like, 'I've jumped over fire!'"

Besides offering a thrilling buzz, obstacle races also serve as a fitness goal for many people. With increasing numbers of people tipping the scales much farther than they'd like, training for an obstacle race provides an incentive to tackle other, more personal, obstacles in their lives. These races serve as innovative, fun, and challenging goals for getting in shape.

Going to the gym five days a week takes discipline, but how accomplished do you feel after yet another session on the elliptical? Obstacle courses provide a total body workout—plus a feeling of satisfaction you just can't find at the gym!

And just as obstacle races can inspire couch potatoes to get up and move, they inspire people facing other personal challenges to push themselves. "We had a blind man complete our entire course in Georgia in 2010 with the assistance of a friend, and I've seen multiple amputees climb over our Cargo Climb obstacle with one arm," Lauren Shield of Warrior Dash recalled.

Bye-Bye, Boring Ultras

Beyond the fact that obstacle races and traditional road races—including 5ks, 10ks, and marathons—cover similar distances and both involve running, the two types of races are more like third cousins than siblings. They may have a common ancestor, but somewhere along the way, one of the relations co-mingled with a rebellious outsider. This encounter introduced some adventurous genes into its DNA—and that's the branch of the family that evolved into obstacle races.

Traditional races are long, slow yawns for a lot of people. As anyone who has ever pounded miles of pavement can attest, road races can be dull affairs that crush your spirit. Aside from an occasional hill or water stop, few features break up the drudgery of the course. Besides, when you finally cross the finish, there's not much to talk about other than your mile splits and how much your knees, hips, and ankles ache. And when you factor in the social media value (after all, have you really done it if you haven't posted it on Facebook?), there's no comparison: a picture of you running down a paved road … or a shot of yourself army crawling through a mud pit with barbed wire stretched inches from your head?

Triathlons take a few steps toward breaking up the monotony, but they swap out one activity—running—for others—biking and swimming. As Tough Mudder's chief marketing officer told the *LA Times*, triathlons "get too nerdy, expensive, and linear." You not only need a lot of expensive equipment—a good bike alone can set you back several hundred (or several thousand) dollars—but you *still* face mind-numbing stretches of doing the same thing.

> **Note**
>
> **Obstacle races are often confused with adventure races. Adventure races are typically multiday affairs in which participants rely on skills such as orienteering and mountaineering to navigate wilderness courses.**

And did we mention the postrace party, complete with live entertainment, food vendors, competitions, and, of course, adult beverages? Competitors swear beer tastes better with mud.

It's All About the Obstacles

Of course, the obstacles and other challenges are what distinguish Rebel Race, Run For Your Lives, and the rest of the obstacle races featured in this book from regular road, trail, and even adventure races. When you're hoisting yourself up and over a wall, plunging into a chest-deep pit of mud, or getting your lactic juices surging on a steep climb while carrying a 5-gallon bucket of rocks, you've left reality behind for awhile. And the beauty of obstacle racing is that no race is ever the same twice. Race organizers are constantly upping the ante by changing the courses and adding new obstacles.

Head over to Chapter 3 to get the scoop on how to conquer the wide variety of obstacles you can expect to encounter.

With a Little Help from Your Friends

Most traditional races and triathlons are solitary endeavors, and even though hundreds of participants compete, they do so as individuals. There's very little interaction among participants as they put their head down, grit their teeth, and put one foot in front of the other … and the other … and the other …. In a road race, it's you, the pavement, and the clock.

Such a scenario contrasts sharply with the vibe at obstacle races, where some race organizers encourage teamwork among participants at every opportunity. Many obstacle races emphasize teamwork and camaraderie even more than winning. In the Muddy Buddy, you must participate in the race with a partner, and you both have to cross the finish—which happens to be strategically placed at the end of a 50-yard-long mud pit—together. In the GORUCK Challenge, your team consists of 29 other people; over the next 8 to 10 hours, you must cooperate with your teammates continually.

Note

> Multiple Spartan race champion Hobie Call gave teamwork a whole new meaning when he tethered himself to his wife, Irene, for the duration of the 2012 Arizona Super Spartan.

According to Sophie Pollitt-Cohen, director of the GORUCK Challenge, the overall challenge GORUCK teams have to solve is being a team and working together. "They start out as 30 strangers, and it takes time to come together—there are 30 personalities at play, and with that can come pride, anxiety," she said. It's the job of the staff leading the team—the Cadre—to put them through missions that by definition make them come together and put all those emotions aside.

One of the problems teams encounter is a member who can't go on, because they are physically or mentally exhausted—or both. "If the person wants to quit in the middle, usually the team simply won't let them. They'll say, 'We're a team, we're going to help you' until the person is convinced to stay," Brian Richardson, Lead Cadre at GORUCK, says. "Other times they've carried an exhausted person for literally miles to make sure they all finish together."

Richardson also reports that, along the same lines as strangers coming together as a team, what he sees now more than ever is the leadership dynamic. During each mission teams are assigned two leaders from within the group. "Many people are either not comfortable leading or being led by someone who has not proven themselves worthy of leading. There can be conflict and a sense of insecurity that can come from being under stress and expected to accomplish the mission," he notes. "This opens a completely new social dilemma that the team must overcome and there is no one absolute solution."

Tough Mudder requires participants to sign a pledge to help "fellow Mudders complete the course" and to "put teamwork and camaraderie before my course time." The pledge comes in handy at the foot of the Everest obstacle (a vertical greased pipe that Mudders must climb), which is very difficult to ascend without a helping hand. "Reminds you why you go to this event with a group," one Mudder told a local newspaper covering an event.

Jane Di Leo, spokesperson for Tough Mudder, says that "We always look at the posters on Facebook. People post, 'I want to run, I don't have a teammate' and you'll see like 50 responses from complete strangers, 'come with us.'"

The whole basis of Tough Mudder is that it's not a race; it's a challenge, with obstacles based on military training—which is all about teamwork, Di Leo pointed out.

Tip

> Want to watch a champion in action? Check out the training videos by the world's top obstacle race athlete, Hobie Call, at conqueranycourse.com.

Sometimes you might start off solo, but find help along the way anyway. Carrie Adams, brand manager for Spartan Race, remembered her first encounter with the 8-foot wall obstacle. "My first race, I ran up a steep incline through mountains and got [to the wall] before the rest of the group. A man came up behind me and just grabbed the back of my jersey and put a hand under my foot and basically threw me over."

Even races that don't allow teams acknowledge that cooperating with fellow athletes can be beneficial. For instance, Run For Your Lives, which doesn't have a team component, admits on its website that it "may be strategically valuable to cooperate with other runners."

Smells Like Team Spirit

Given the cooperative nature of the majority of the races, it only makes sense that many of them encourage participants to join as teams. The Civilian Military Combine (CMC) has a team division that allows competitors to band together with two or three others.

Being on a team can certainly up the camaraderie quotient during the race. And if your teammates live near you, having a partner to train with can help you stick with a training regimen. It's no secret that being accountable to someone else helps keep the couch potato urges at bay, because nobody likes to admit that they're staying home to watch *Mad Men* reruns rather than hitting the gym or the track.

Check out the following table to see how each obstacle race handles teams.

Obstacle Race Team Requirements

Obstacle Race	Team Info
Civilian Military Combine (CMC)	Three- or four-person teams; team division scoring based on average time (the course) and number of reps (The PIT); team members don't have to finish the course together
Columbia Muddy Buddy & Run Series	Two-person teams; teammates are required to finish course together
GORUCK Challenge	You can register with others as a team, but teams are absorbed into the larger 30-person team
Merrell Down and Dirty	No team division
Mudathlon	Five-person or more team; top five times are averaged for scoring
Rebel Race	Teams of any size welcome, but no team scoring
Rugged Maniac	Teams of any size welcome, but no team scoring
Run For Your Lives	No team division
Spartan	Four- or more person teams for the Sprint, Super Spartan, and Beast; top four times are averaged for team scoring
SuperHero Scramble	No team division
The Survival Race	No team division
Tough Mudder	Teams of any size welcome
Warrior Dash	No team division

Flying Solo

Nobody is going to hold it against you if you're not into the whole team spirit thing. Lone wolves have their pick of obstacle races, too. You just need to choose your event wisely. Go ahead and cross the GORUCK Challenge and the Muddy Buddy off your "potential race" list right now. The GORUCK Challenge is all about teamwork, and you can't enter the Muddy Buddy without, well, a buddy. Tough Mudder talks a lot about teamwork and camaraderie, but you can go it alone if you really want to. All of the other races have individual divisions so that you can be the mud-stained star of your own obstacle race reality show.

Testing Your Mettle

Obstacle courses aren't for the faint of heart. An article in *Maclean's* counted 35 participants finishing a Spartan Death Race out of the 155 who started. But the Death Race is certainly at the extreme end of the danger spectrum. Amit Nar, founder of Rebel Race, shared some more encouraging statistics: on average, 95 percent finish the 5k race and 85 percent finish the 15k.

What makes the difference? Maybe it's all in your head, as Sophie Pollitt-Cohen, director of GORUCK Challenge, seems to attest: "We say it's all mental, and it really is. As a friend once responded when I asked him if I should train—'will getting punched in the face train you to get punched in the face really hard? Probably.' It's nearly impossible to be perfectly prepared because so much of the Challenge is about pushing through—through being cold, wet, tired, worried about letting your team down."

GORUCK's Brian Richardson said he generally doesn't suggest any one plan for preparing. "The best I can offer is accept that there will be times when you will want to quit, and when you physically cannot continue. Know that the person to the left and right of you are going through the same thing. Keep going for them, for the team, for the mission."

The courses are designed to push you mentally. Jane Di Leo of Tough Mudder pointed to the event's Electroshock Therapy obstacle—a field of live wires that can deliver up to 10,000 volts painful enough to drop a big man. And just beyond the field? The finish line.

The event has welcomed injured soldiers, cancer survivors, double amputees, paralympians, and people who just want to get fit or lose weight. "So many people use [Tough Mudder] as a turning point in their lives," she said. "We had a guy from Walter Reed [military hospital], who said step one was walking again, step two was doing Tough Mudder. The idea of overcoming obstacles is what Tough Mudder is all about."

Obstacle races are meant to get people thinking of fitness in a new way, to get you motivated and looking forward to something that feels like a real accomplishment.

"We want to be an event that is so tough that in a few years, a guy will be able to go up to a girl in a bar and say, 'I'm a Tough Mudder' and she'll be impressed," Di Leo said. "We want it to be something people will brag about."

Finding the Right Fit

Not every obstacle race is a good fit for every individual. Some races are just too extreme for beginners, and some are beyond the abilities of many experienced racers. The Spartan Death Race, with its grueling climbs, sadistic challenges, and marathon distances can crush the spirit of all but the most hardened competitors. And those same sadomasochists attracted to extreme races might scoff at the thought of donning a costume and completing a "mere" 3.2-mile course peppered with wall climbs, giant slides, and monkey bars.

Tip

Most obstacle races have Facebook pages, which are a great place to see more photos of the races, get a feel for their vibe, and find out what participants have to say about them. Just be aware that the races can ban users who post negative comments, so you're likely only going to see positive feedback.

You should also take your personality into account when picking a race. According to Junyong Pak, one of the world's top obstacle racers, "Spartan is a very, very serious race, timed race. You against the clock. [Spartan's] obstacles are generally more focused toward physical abilities."

Pak also points out that, "Tough Mudder's obstacles are more psychologically challenging …. Generally you're just trying to finish the event."

And then there are what Pak refers to as the "gateway" obstacle races, such as the Muddy Buddy and Warrior Dash. These less-challenging courses are a way for people who might be intimidated by the seriousness of the Spartan races or daunted by the obstacles at Tough Mudder to give obstacle racing a try.

We've done the hard work of picking races that even seasoned competitors—at least the ones with a good sense of humor—would find challenging enough to take on. In other words, you won't be reading about lame obstacles that encompass running around plastic pink flamingoes.

When picking out races, don't make the mistake of thinking that just because it's shorter, it's easier. According to Hobie Call, "Some of the toughest races I've done are the sprints because they're so obstacle intense. Run a little bit, obstacle, run a little bit, obstacle. So the longer the race, the more running you're going to be doing between obstacles. So if you like running, do the longer race. Obstacles in a 12-mile race aren't any harder or more numerous than in a 3-mile race."

For Camaraderie and Fun

Every race draws a sizeable contingent of folks who just want to have a good time. You can usually spot these people right away, because they're the ones wearing the costumes, mugging for the camera, and making a day (or even a weekend) out of the event.

"One of my first events, there was a group of guys in spandex dressed as pigs," Jane Di Leo of Tough Mudder said, laughing. Warrior Dash has seen a group of racers in Arizona dress in Hawaiian luau attire and carry a keg, and another group lugging a mini refrigerator through the entire course and over the obstacles.

For a Good Cause

Charity has been an integral part of obstacle racing. For example, Tough Mudder has raised nearly $3 million for the Wounded Warrior Project, a charity that helps soldiers hurt during combat. The following table lists the charities each race described in this book is connected with.

Obstacle Race Charitable Support

Obstacle Race	Charity
Civilian Military Combine (CMC)	LIVESTRONG, Operation Homefront, and Heroes of Tomorrow

continues

continued

Obstacle Race	Charity
Columbia Muddy Buddy & Run Series	The Challenged Athletes Foundation
GORUCK Challenge	Green Beret Foundation
Mudathlon	Location-specific charities for each event
Rebel Race	Participants can choose from a number of different charities to donate to
Rugged Maniac	The Fisher House Foundation
Run For Your Lives	American Red Cross
Spartan Races	Home for Our Troops and Help for Our Heroes
SuperHero Scramble	Forgotten Soldiers Outreach and Kids in Distress
The Survival Race	Donates $50 to each volunteer's favorite charity
Tough Mudder	Wounded Warrior Project
Warrior Dash	St. Jude Children's Research Hospital

The Nuts and Bolts: Registering for the Race

You can register for all the races featured in this book on the race websites listed in "The Down and Dirty" sidebars for each race in Chapter 2. Some races also have booths at the races where spectators caught up in the fun can register for future races.

Races like to fill their capacity early, and they often offer discounts for early registration. Still, the races aren't cheap, and you do get what you pay for; more expensive events are usually higher in quality. Expect to pay between $50 and $160 to enter an obstacle race. Note that most race entries are nonrefundable and nontransferable. At many races, you actually register for a particular wave, or start time. Late morning waves tend to fill early, leaving the early morning and afternoon waves for later registrants. Races organize their events by waves in order to minimize the wait time at the obstacles.

Tip

Register for the earliest heat, or wave, you can stomach. Not only will you avoid the higher temps later in the day, but you will get the course when it's fresh. Some of the races can draw 10,000 to 20,000 runners over a single weekend, which can take a serious toll on the course.

In addition to a spot in the race and access to the postrace party, your entry fee typically gets you the following swag: a T-shirt; a finisher medal, patch, or headband or hat; and one free beer for participants 21 and older.

At some point between the time that you register for the race and when you queue up at the start, every race is going to require you to sign a release form containing all sorts of legal niceties. If you squint really hard, you'll see that it's a death waiver, releasing the race from any responsibility should you be injured or die on the course.

Take a deep breath. And if you follow the training program in this book, you'll be in great shape to conquer the course. Just sign the waiver, and make sure that your health and life insurance policies are paid up through race day.

Chapter 2

The Races

On summer nights when I was young, I used to play a game with the kids in my neighborhood that we called Bloody Murder. I've long since forgotten the rules—it was some type of nighttime hide-and-go-seek—but I can still recall the overall experience with surprising clarity: the exhilaration of the chase, all of my senses heightened by the chest-pounding fear of what lurked in the dark, and the surge of relief, joy, and victory as I made the final push to the safe zone, located 20 feet above the ground on a limb of a big oak tree.

My mom, after calling me in for the night, would march me straight to the shower and order me to clean off the dirt that was caked on my knees, hands, and elbows. Although a good scrubbing erased the grime, all the soap in the world couldn't wash away the grin plastered on my face. After toweling off, I crawled into bed utterly exhausted, still savoring the pure joy of the evening.

My childhood experience is far from singular. Most adults played such games as kids and had as much fun as I did doing it. But more rare is our ability to recapture those moments as grown-ups. How long has it been since you've done something that was so pure, so intense, so fun, so challenging, and so frightening—all at the same time?

Or for that matter, how long has it been since you've gotten dirty? I'm not talking about the kind of dirty you get when you're landscaping your yard or cleaning out your basement. No, I'm talking grit-in-your-teeth and mud-clogging-your-hair-follicles filthy. Like when you were a kid and you had the option of taking the shortcut through the swamp or going the long way around it. For kids, high and dry loses every time.

To quote multiple Spartan Race champion Hobie Call, the races I describe in this chapter give you "a chance to be a kid again." They are an adult playground, complete with monkey bars, rope climbs, and mud pits.

But these races aren't mere kids' stuff. As a matter of fact, some of them make grown men and women cry. As one race participant put it, they turn you inside out and make you face your biggest fears. Anytime you have to sign a death waiver, you better ask, "What am I getting myself into?" And although only a few people have actually died while attempting these races, if you spend any time around veterans of some of the more challenging versions of these races, you'll hear plenty of tales of participants puking their guts out, getting scraped by barbed wire, and having their egos beaten into submission.

As one race's motto puts it: "You'll know at the finish line." And that's what makes obstacle racing so exhilarating.

About the Races

For each event I provide a brief description of the course, its obstacles, the type of atmosphere at the event, and advice for tackling some of the most difficult aspects of the challenge.

Some races are all about having a good time, with a smidge of competition thrown in to spice things up. Other races take competition to new levels of extreme. Most races, however, fall comfortably in the middle, managing to offer a serious competition without taking themselves too seriously. And although I rate each race by its overall level of difficulty, don't let the rating scare you away from a particular race if you really want to do it—all but the most challenging are generally quite inclusive.

I review a wide spectrum of races, but you can rest assured that any race I cover provides a quality, safe (relatively speaking—these are physically demanding courses, after all), and rewarding experience for participants. You won't find any flimflam obstacles or fly-by-night race operators described in these pages.

I also provide you with some down and dirty details about each race. These include:

Levels of Difficulty

Couch potatoes welcome!   Easiest; minimal training necessary to have a good time

I didn't say it would be easy   Moderate difficulty; perfect for weekend warriors

Cringe and bear it   Very physically challenging; train a minimum of six weeks

Sick and twisted   Very physically *and* psychologically challenging; train a minimum of eight weeks plus have competed in less difficult races in order to build mental toughness

Off the charts   'Nuff said

How Dirty Will You Get?

First-degree dirty   Postrace shower optional

Second-degree dirty   How dirty you get depends on how much you like playing in mud

Third-degree dirty   You'll have to do more than rinse and repeat to get rid of all this grime

I tried my best to include the most up-to-date race information for 2013, but races are always adding new locations, so check their website to find out exact locations.

Finally, I caution you to keep in mind that courses vary significantly from location to location and from year to year. The terrain often dictates how the obstacles are presented. Many of the races have general obstacles they use in all races but add other surprise obstacles based around the unique features of the course.

Civilian Military Combine (CMC)

The CMC is about as red, white, and blue as obstacle races get, drawing armed forces personnel and folks who just want to see if they have the right stuff to compete in a military-style competition. Unique to the CMC is The PIT, a challenge preceding the obstacle run in which participants are judged on the number of reps they do in four timed lifting events. If you do too many reps, you might not have any strength left for the obstacle course.

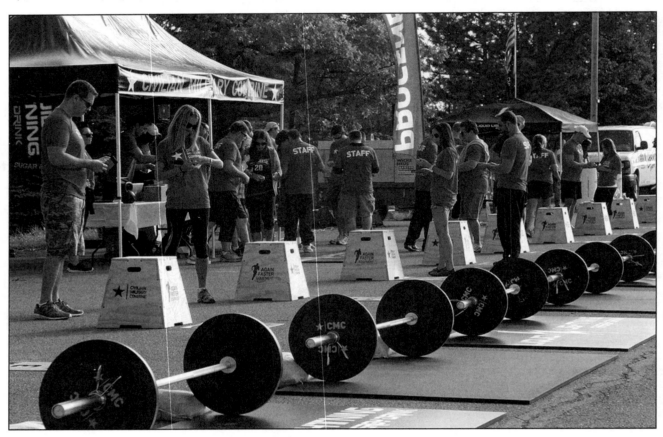

(Photo courtesy of Nuvision Action Image)

The Down and Dirty

Locations: Bryce Resort, VA; Camelback, PA

Course: Four judged lifting events in The PIT followed by a 5- to 7-mile mountain course with 25 military obstacles, including multiple water features

Level of Difficulty: Cringe and bear it

How Dirty Will You Get? Third-degree dirty

How Many Finish? 85 percent

Postrace Activities: None

Website: civilianmilitarycombine.com

Event Atmosphere

You won't find anyone dressed up as a superhero for this event, but you might run alongside a real hero or two—military or former military personnel who have put their lives on the line for their country. Military-lite might be the best way to describe the intense, "Ooh-rah!" atmosphere here. Many people participate as part of a team, and patriotism and camaraderie among teammates prevail.

What to Expect

You can participate as a team of three or four competitors (scoring is based on total number of reps in The PIT and lowest average race time) or as an individual. You must complete all PIT challenges and obstacles in order to be considered for scoring. Because these events take place at ski resorts, plan to climb a lot of hills.

The Obstacles

The PIT: You have 90 seconds at each station to do as many reps as you dare of thrusters (front squat into overhead press; 75 pounds for men, 44 pounds for women), burpees, box jumps (20 inches), and kettlebell swings (40 pounds for men, 20 pounds for women).

Other obstacles making an appearance at the CMC may include:

Sandbag/Log Carry: Carry a heavy sandbag up a hill

Water Crossing: Run through knee-deep water

Over Unders: Climb over and under log obstacles

Hurdles: Jump over hurdles along the course

Incline Wall: Pull yourself up and over a wall

Ranger Ropes: Make like a monkey and cross a rope strung over a water feature

Hay Bale Mountain: Conquer a pile of hay bales

Low Crawl: Crawl through water under barbed wire

Downhill Water Chute: Enjoy the ride!

Cargo Net Climb: Clamber up a rope net

Balance Beam River Crossing: Avoid falling into the river as you walk across a narrow beam

Expert Advice

One key to succeeding in the CMC is figuring out how many reps you can do in The PIT without tiring yourself too much for the ensuing race and obstacle course. The PIT weights are actually pretty light; it's the reps that can kill you. If you do too many kettlebells, for example, you might not have enough arm strength left to pull yourself over the incline wall or hay bale mountain. Similarly, too many box jumps will make the hurdles appear to grow in height before your eyes.

One of the best ways to train for the rigors of this event is to practice each PIT exercise in advance and then do a run. Increase your reps and your distance in the weeks leading up to the race. While training, force yourself to run on hilly terrain. If you only train on level ground, 7 miles will feel like double that distance when you have to run a course that has several up-and-down hills, so the sooner you get used to it, the better.

GORUCK Challenge

Organizers are careful to stress that this is a *challenge,* not a *race.* And although physical stamina is certainly required, perhaps the bigger trial of this military-inspired event is working as a team to accomplish your goal. Along the way you must use your problem-solving skills, leadership, and strength to complete the course under the orders of a badass cadre (drill sergeant) while carrying a weighted rucksack around a city.

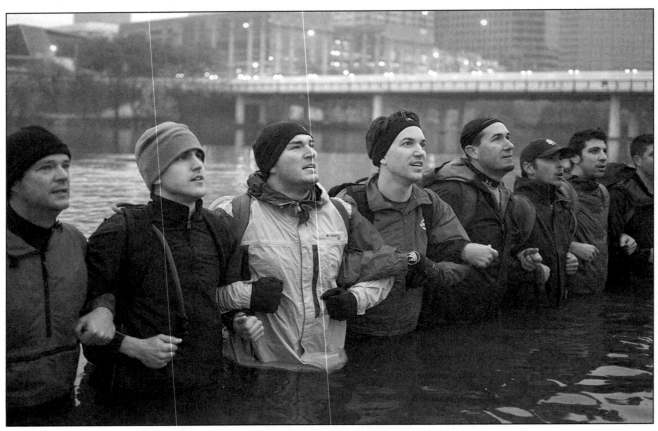

(Photo courtesy of the GORUCK Challenge)

The Down and Dirty

Locations: More than 60 U.S. cities and 7 international locations

Course: A 15- to 20-mile urban "tour" of the host city, including famous landmarks and sights, such as the steps of the Philadelphia Art Museum (think *Rocky*), the Brooklyn Bridge, and the Pacific Ocean

Level of Difficulty: Cringe and bear it

How Dirty Will You Get? Second-degree dirty

How Many Finish? 98 percent

Postrace Activities: None

Website: goruckchallenge.com

Event Atmosphere

The official drink of the GORUCK is beer, so you know these folks don't take themselves too seriously. However, when you're out on a challenge in the middle of the night with a 40-pound rucksack on your back, a cadre who is ordering you to drop and give him 20 *after* you've carried a heavy log for the past three hours, and a teammate who is simultaneously retching and weeping, you realize that you're going to have to *earn* that beer.

What to Expect

Expect an urban tour on steroids run by a drill sergeant. Although this is a military-style challenge, the majority of participants have no military experience, and 10 percent are women. Plan to spend 8 to 10 hours on the course, often throughout the night.

The Obstacles

The GORUCK offers no obstacles in the traditional sense of the word, although all participants must carry a weighted GORUCK rucksack throughout the event. (You must purchase one if you don't already own one.) Your cadre orders you to perform exercises such as crab walks, fence climbs, low crawls and, of course, lengthy runs—all while wearing your rucksack. Missions typically include carrying a heavy log for several hours—no easy feat when your teammates are of varying heights and fitness levels.

Expert Advice

Endurance and functional strength training will serve you well for this event, but much of your success depends on everyone in the group putting the team before their individual needs. If you want to succeed, you need to set your ego aside and work with others to achieve difficult goals.

Mudathlon

Mudathlon puts participants in the mud as much as possible, with a variety of mud and water obstacles dotting its 3-mile, country-themed courses.

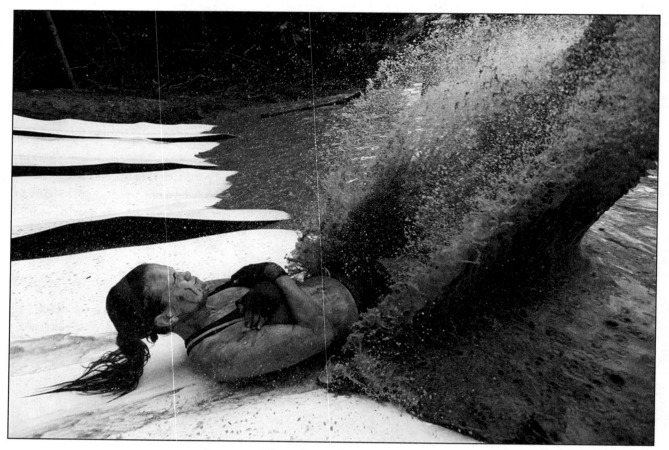

(Photo by Nick Graham)

The Down and Dirty

Locations: Northern Kentucky, Indianapolis, Northwest Indiana, and Cincinnati

Course: 3-mile off-road course with 40 obstacles

Level of Difficulty: I didn't say it would be easy

How Dirty Will You Get? Third-degree dirty

How Many Finish? 95 percent

Postrace Activities: Postrace party where the beer is flowing, the brats are smoking, and the live music is jamming

Website: mudathlon.com

Event Atmosphere

An event featuring lots of camaraderie and a postrace partylike atmosphere. More than half of all participants compete as part of a team, and many hang out afterward and make it an all-day event. Slightly more than half of the participants are female, and the average age is 33. Costumes are encouraged.

What to Expect

If you can't complete an obstacle within a reasonable amount of time, a course marshal will ask you to bypass it in order to avoid bottlenecks. But once you skip an obstacle, you're out of the running for an award.

The Obstacles

A few of our favorite Mudathlon obstacles include:

Shifty Spools: Climb up and over two huge wooden spools

Cargo Cling and Climb: Climb a cargo net and jump 10 feet down off the other side

Paintball Ambush: Avoid getting splattered by paintball gun–toting rednecks (to complement the country theme)

Hay: Climb up and over 7-foot bales of hay

The Cricketed Creek Crossing: Sprint 100 yards through a creek

The Slide: Slide 30 feet down a muddy hill into a muddy water pit

Mucking Mud Pit: Crawl through a 100-yard mud pit face first

Sludge Run: Slog through the mud

Tunnel of Terror: Crawl through a pipe

The Wall: Conquer a wooden barricade

Expert Advice

Race waves head out every 15 minutes and include all ability levels, so if you want to avoid waiting in line at obstacles, get an early lead in your heat.

Columbia Muddy Buddy Ride & Run Series

Truth in advertising prevails for this race: you will get muddy. And you do need a buddy. But if you and your partner are okay getting a little sludge up your nostrils, you'll have a blast in this popular, family-friendly series of events.

The Muddy Buddy Run is a team event in which two runners pair up and complete the course together. In the Muddy Buddy Bike & Run, teammates share a single bike, with partners alternating between biking and running the course, switching roles at each obstacle. Bring the kids along and enter them in the Mini Mud Buddy (ages 4 to 11), featuring a short obstacle course leading into the mud pit.

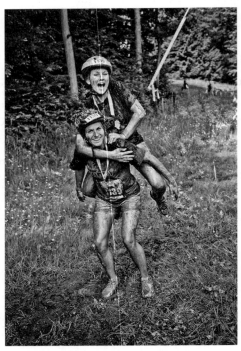

(Photo courtesy of Muddy Buddy)

The Down and Dirty

Locations: Portland, OR; Boulder, CO; Chicago, IL; Nashville, TN; Richmond, VA; Atlanta, GA; Austin, TX; San Jose, CA

Muddy Buddy Run Course: Well-marked double-wide trails traversing 3 to 4 miles and interspersed with 8 to 10 obstacles, including a 50-foot mud pit leading into the finish that you must crawl through with your buddy

Muddy Buddy Run & Bike Course: 6- to 7-mile course and 5 obstacles, including the infamous mud pit

Level of Difficulty: Couch potatoes welcome!

How Dirty Will You Get? Third-degree dirty

How Many Finish? 98 percent

Postrace Activities: Postrace party with food and two free beers (must be 21 or older for alcohol)

Website: muddybuddy.com

Event Atmosphere

Costumes, lively music, and an overall mellow vibe make this race one of the most family friendly out there. Many participants put more effort into their costumes than they do training for the event, which pays off for them at the prerace costume contest.

The divisions are male, female, co-ed, and Beast; in the latter division, teammates must weigh a combined minimum of 420 pounds. Weigh-ins take place during the awards ceremony for the Beast division, and teams coming in under 420 pounds are good-naturedly booed off the stage. Nearly half the field is made up of co-ed teams, and more than one guy has "popped the question" to his gal in the mud pit.

What to Expect

If you don't think competition should involve lots of laughs, goofy costumes, and music during the race, then this one isn't for you.

The Obstacles

Obstacles are designed to be fun rather than intimidating. But if an obstacle scares you, you can simply run around it, no questions asked and no penalties imposed. In addition to a number of surprise obstacles, expect the following:

Not So Low Wall: Grab a cargo hold to help pull yourself over the 7-foot wall

Running from the Law: Make your way over multiple 4-foot walls

Beware The Frog Maze: Find your way out of the fog-shrouded maze

Steeplechase Hurdles: Jump over the hurdles between each obstacle

Marine Assault Inflatable: Navigate a watery obstacle in which you must go over and under horizontal logs, traverse incline walls, and make your way through tubes

Slide For Your Life: Grab hold of the cargo net to make your way up the 20-foot wall leading to a slide

Mr. Frog's Buddy Blockade: Grab hold of the muddy ropes to pull yourself up and over a 12-foot wall and down the ladder on the other side

The Mud Pit: Trudge your way through a 50-foot-long mud pit

Expert Advice

Although the Bike & Run's buddy system is about as straightforward as these sorts of things get (leapfrog your partner between biking and running; make the transition at the obstacle), people tend to get flustered in the heat of competition. That's why experienced Muddy Buddies recommend that bikers yell to their partner as they pass them by, so the runner knows that the bike is waiting for them at the next obstacle and looks for it right away rather than waiting needlessly.

More tips: decorate your bicycle so that it stands out from the crowd, and decide ahead of time to always leave it in a certain location in the transition area. No need to make finding your bike an extra obstacle.

The Rebel Race

One part race, two parts party, particularly if you pitch a tent at the on-site campground (for many races) and make a weekend of it.

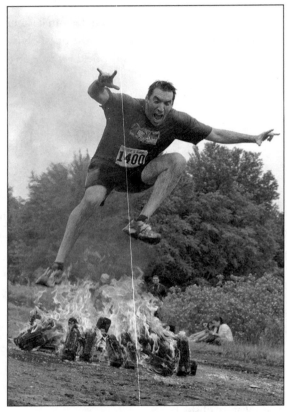

(Photo courtesy of Oz Sports Photography)

The Down and Dirty

Locations: Eight locations throughout the United States including Atlanta, GA; Dallas, TX; Central Texas; Maryland; and Indiana

Course: 5k (3.2 miles) and 15k (9.6 miles) trail race in which terrain varies by location and can be very hilly

Level of Difficulty: I didn't say it would be easy

How Dirty Will You Get? Third-degree dirty

How Many Finish? 95 percent finish the 5k; 85 percent finish the 15k

Postrace Activities: Party including one free beer (for racers) with plenty more beer and tasty barbecue available for purchase; other events include tug of war, a mechanical bull, and the Muddy Dance Party

Website: rebelrace.com

Event Atmosphere

Each rebel is competing to be first to finish the race, but they're willing to help each other during the course. You'll see a lot of teams work to get up the Hell at the Himalayas because the hill is steep and extremely muddy, so people keep slipping. After the race, it's a party atmosphere. Every rebel is in a good mood because he or she finished and gets to bask in the glory with a free beer, music, and barbecue.

What to Expect

Although a good race for first-timers, this race is more difficult than some other popular entry-level races. The Rebel gets people from all walks of life, from young athletes in their 20s to people going through a midlife crisis who want to prove they've still got it. Many people run with friends.

The Obstacles

Obstacles vary by location but typically include the mud pit, balance beam, fire leap, slide, ditch crossing, hay bale climb, rope wall, net climb, mud pits under barbed wire, over-and-under walls, and the tunnel scramble. Participants list the following obstacles in order of difficulty:

Rebellious Roping: Rope climb over water

Fast Twitch Tires: High-knee your way through a tire course

Clamber the Cargo: Climb a cargo net

Hay Dude: Clamber over a massive hay bale pyramid

Gamble with Gravity: Pull yourself over a wall using a rope

Ninja Turtle Sewer: Make your way through tunnels

Unleashed Endurance: Go over and under logs in the water

Hell at the Himalayas: Conquer a mountain made of mud

Military Mud Pit: Crawl through a mud pit strung with barbed wire

Slimy Slope Slide: Hop on and slide down

Expert Advice

Rebel Race organizers, tongue in cheek, suggest digging a mud pit in your neighbor's yard to bathe in, but founder Amit Nar had some more practical advice. "If you're better prepared for the course, you can do more and have more fun doing it. Work on endurance, forearm strength, stuff like that. If you can't get through the obstacle, you didn't prepare enough, you're not fit enough."

He suggests running 5 miles at least three days a week, with half of the run including sprints up steep hills. Add jump roping for an hour five days a week. "That can do so much for endurance and the sprints will give you speed," he said. Nar also recommends eight minutes of abdominal exercises each night, including leg lifts and crunches. Finally, do circuit weights, with three sets for each part of the body. "Forearm exercises are key. You need the forearms for the wall, really, and the roping. For the crawling obstacles, you need good abs."

Rugged Maniac

Numerous, well-constructed obstacles and varied terrain contribute to the overall quality of the Rugged Maniac, a race that manages to gracefully tread the balance beam between grit-your-teeth-and-growl competitive and laugh-so-hard-you-spit-out-your-beer spirited.

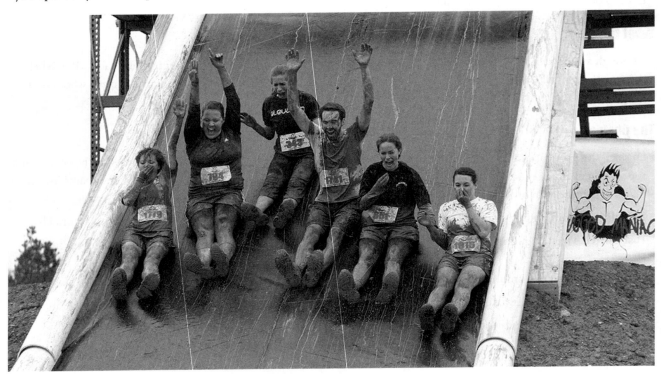

(Photo courtesy of Rugged Races LLC)

The Down and Dirty

Locations: 14 U.S. locations, including several along the East Coast

Course: Flat to very hilly 5k course that varies by location; each course features at least 20 obstacles

Level of Difficulty: I didn't say it would be easy

How Dirty Will You Get? Third-degree dirty

How Many Finish? 90 percent

Postrace Activities: Party with live music, food, and plenty of beer

Website: ruggedmaniac.com

Event Atmosphere

They come for the obstacles, but they stay for the party. Or is it the other way around? In any case, expect a good mix of serious and just-for-fun participants tackling the course and lingering long after to sip beer, swap stories, and savor the satisfaction of crossing the finish line. About half of the participants are female, making this race more gender balanced than many races.

Note: Spectators must purchase tickets.

What to Expect

You need to be in excellent shape to come out near the top in this race, which features quality obstacles and a fairly large contingent of competitive racers. If you view the race as a mere prelude to the postrace party, bring a change of clothes (shoes included), a good attitude, and moderate physical stamina. Races held at ski resorts (Wilmot, Wisconsin; Weston, Montana; and Turners Falls, Minnesota) are the most difficult due to the steep terrain.

The Obstacles

You can skip obstacles, but then you'll be disqualified from any time-based prizes. Obstacles vary by location but typically include barbed wire crawls, fire leaps, tunnel crawls, floating barriers, balancing beams, pools of water, barricades, cargo net climb, scrambles, swinging pendulums, slides, tire jungle, wall climbs, and over-and-under barriers. Here are some of our favorites:

Bounding Maniac: Run through this water obstacle as it's best crossed at full speed

Rugged Mud: Crawl under low-slung barbed wire through mud

Balancing Maniac: Cross thin, bouncy planks suspended over water

Big Tunnels: Duck to walk through the tunnel

Tire Jungle: Move over, under, and through tires on the ground, tires in the air, tires everywhere

Maniac Barricades: Climb over walls 3 to 7 feet high

Little Tunnels: Crawl through pipes

Prometheus Leap: Jump over fiery obstacles

Expert Advice

The obstacles at the Rugged Maniac are generally very doable. It's the running that's going to hurt, particularly on the more hilly courses. If you want to come out near the top in this course, you should be able to run 3 miles without stopping. On race day, position yourself near the front of your heat.

Oh, and wait until *after* the race to start drinking beer.

Run For Your Lives

A zombie-apocalypse atmosphere permeates this 5k (3.2 miles) obstacle race. There's little doubt that you'll be able to overcome the obstacles and finish the race. The question is whether you can evade the zombies, who chase you down and try to steal the three flags you're given at the start. If by some spooky twist of fate you cross the finish line without any flags, you're considered one of the "undead" and don't qualify for any prizes.

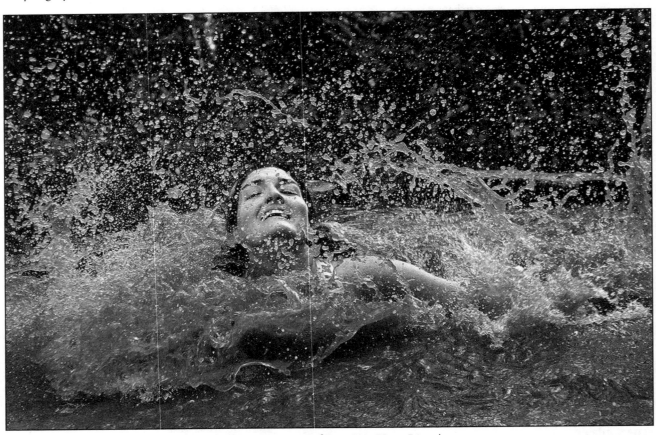

(Photo courtesy of Run For Your Lives)

The Down and Dirty

Locations: Massachusetts, Indiana, Maryland, Texas, Colorado, Southern California, Minnesota, Florida, Washington, Pennsylvania, Missouri

Course: 5k (3.2 miles) over varied terrain with 10 to 12 man-made and natural obstacles, plus zombies

Level of Difficulty: Couch potatoes welcome!

How Dirty Will You Get? Third-degree dirty

How Many Finish? 98 percent

Postrace Activities: Apocalypse Party featuring food, music, beer, and prizes

Website: runforyourlives.com

Event Atmosphere

This fun-filled race has enough challenges to appeal to seasoned racers, but also offers a laid-back vibe that puts first-time runners at ease. The event also attracts zombie fanatics, making for one of the more unique experiences on the obstacle race circuit.

Note: Nonrunners must purchase a Spectator Pass to watch the event; the pass also gives them access to the Apocalypse Party, which features food, music, and prizes.

What to Expect

You must have moderate physical stamina and be able to evade zombies—costumed volunteers hidden along the course who pop out to try to steal your flags.

The Obstacles

Race organizers closely guard the course and the obstacles for each race location, adding to the mystery and the challenge of the event. You can skip an obstacle, but then you're considered a zombie and are ineligible for prizes. Here are some obstacles you're likely to encounter:

Cargo Net: Grab the rope netting and climb up and over this 15-foot wall

Wall Climb: Climb up one side and slide down the other

Hay Bale Maze: Avoid the zombies lurking throughout this maze of bales

Over-and-Unders: Climb over and duck under a series of obstacles

Hay Bale Pyramid: Climb over a pile of—you guessed it!—hay bales

Terrible Tubes: Crawl through pipes

Water Pit: Slide down a slick, muddy pit into a pool of water

Expert Advice

Past participants recommend running with a group to spread the risk of being caught by a zombie. Other tips include spinning as zombies approach (making it harder for them to grab the flags), and even disguising yourself as a zombie as a form of camouflage.

Spartan Beast

Unlike some other events I cover in this book, the Spartan series doesn't shy away from calling its events *races,* and yes, the Spartan folks are keeping score. The serious competitors who enter the Beast like it that way.

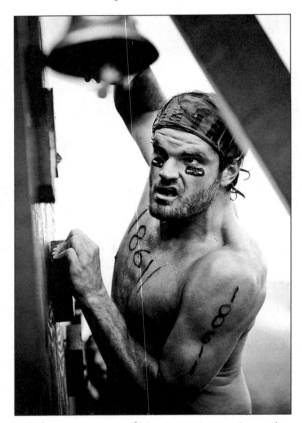

(Photo courtesy of Nuvision Action Image)

The Down and Dirty

Locations: Approximately eight events in the United States and Canada

Course: Grueling 10+-mile course

Level of Difficulty: Sick and twisted

How Dirty Will You Get? Third-degree dirty

How Many Finish? 50 to 60 percent

Postrace Activities: Free postrace festivities featuring live bands or DJs either on-site (with food vendors) or at a nearby club

Website: spartanrace.com/spartan-beast-obstacle-course-race.html

Event Atmosphere

Participants in this event typically train very hard and take the race very seriously. The atmosphere is family friendly.

Note: Spectators must pay to attend the event at most venues.

What to Expect

The course is longer. The barbed wire is lower. The pain is more intense. The terrain is more grueling. Expect everything to be more challenging than in the Spartan Sprint and the Super Spartan.

The Obstacles

Unlike some other obstacle races, Spartan doesn't let you skip obstacles without paying a price. And the legal tender is burpees—10 to 30 per obstacle that you skip. Furthermore, you are strongly encouraged to at least try to overcome the obstacle before giving up and doing the burpees instead.

Spartan doesn't reveal in advance what obstacles any particular race features, but they do have the following staples in their obstacle repertoire:

Leap of Faith: Leap over a flaming bale of hay

The Mud Pit: Cross a muddy trench

Mt. Impossible: Climb an 8-foot wall

Heroes Spear Throw: Throw a spear at a target

Dark Tunnel: Crawl through a mud-covered tunnel

The Fallen: Fend off Spartan warriors armed with padded "jousting" clubs

Enemies Trap: Climb a cargo net

Slippery Victory: Climb a greased-up 12-foot slippery wall built at a 45-degree angle

Barbed Crawl: Crawl under barbed wire

Expert Advice

Because of the length of this race, you should make sure that you are prepared to run long distances—often over very tough and hilly terrain—between obstacles. People who are looking for a more obstacle-dense course should opt for the Spartan Sprint instead.

Spartan Death Race

You find out just how far you can push yourself in this sick and twisted event in which race organizers encourage you to withdraw as soon as you register. Journalist and one-time participant Mark Jenkins called it a "demented sufferfest"; he dropped out midway through the race, but he wasn't alone. Fewer than one of every four participants stumble across the finish line—and that's 24 to 48 hours and 40 miles after they start. Spartan recently added a Winter Death Race to its offerings, generously providing competitors two chances to die each year.

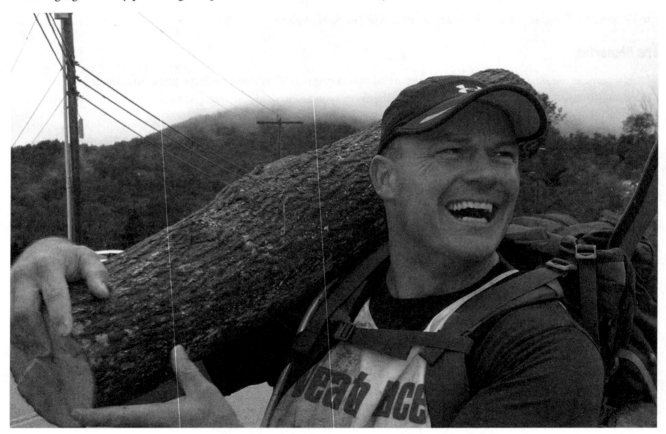

(Photo courtesy of Nuvision Action Image)

The Down and Dirty

Location: Pittsfield, VT

Course: Mountainous terrain covering marathon lengths

Level of Difficulty: Off the charts

How Dirty Will You Get? Third-degree dirty

How Many Finish? Way less than 25 percent

Postrace Activities: Crawling to your car

Website: youmaydie.com

Event Atmosphere

Navy SEAL hell week condensed into one helluva long day (or two). This highly competitive challenge takes on a team feeling as participants bond through mutual suffering, encouraging fellow racers to hang in there as they pass by. Elite endurance athletes elevate to superhero status in this event as they push themselves beyond mental and physical barriers that leave the rest of us on (what's left of) our knees.

What to Expect

You might die—but only after enduring multiple mind games and back-busting challenges that make you question your sanity for ever having entered this race. Expect earlier-than-planned starts (just to get you rattled from the get-go), being told to lug around heavy equipment that you never use, and completing more hill climbs than you can shake a titanium knee joint at.

You are allowed a support crew, whose job is to shove energy gels and orange slices into your mouth and to witness your suffering.

The Obstacles

Expect anywhere from 15 to 20 challenges that involve mind games, insane climbs, tortuous carries, and hellish challenges like memorizing a Bible verse, hiking to the top of the mountain, and reciting the verse; if you miss a single word of the recitation, you have to do it all over again … which might be a good time to start praying.

Participants in the 2012 Winter Death Race suffered through 3,000 burpees, two sessions of Bikram yoga in a room heated to 120°F, and lengthy submersions in freezing-cold water.

Expert Advice

Don't do it.

Okay, okay … if you're really into this thing, make sure you're in peak physical and mental shape and follow this advice from the pros: pace yourself. Start out slow and don't feel like you have to run every hill. Get plenty of rest in advance, and make sure that you are thoroughly hydrated.

Oh, one more thing: make sure your health insurance policy is up to date.

Spartan Sprint

The Spartan Sprint is the easiest of the races in the Spartan series, making it the most approachable event for newcomers. Many people who "graduate" from the Sprint go on to attempt more difficult Spartan races, such as the Super Spartan and the Spartan Beast.

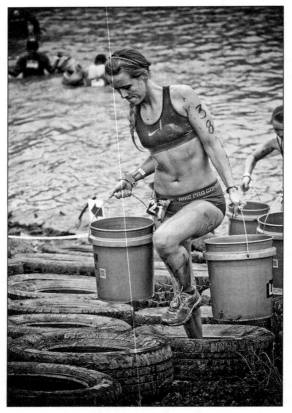

(Photo courtesy of Nuvision Action Image)

The Down and Dirty

Locations: Throughout the United States and Canada

Course: 5k trail race with 10 or more obstacles

Level of Difficulty: I didn't say it would be easy

How Dirty Will You Get? Third-degree dirty

How Many Finish? 90 percent

Postrace Activities: Postrace party featuring food, music, and beer

Website: spartanrace.com/spartan-sprint-obstacle-course-race.html

Event Atmosphere

Expect a family-friendly, inclusive atmosphere and plenty of spectators. More than three fourths of the racers in the Spartan series are between the ages of 20 and 39. Participants take the race very seriously while typically maintaining a high level of sportsmanship and camaraderie.

Note: Spectators must pay to attend the event at most venues.

What to Expect

Brand manager Carrie Adams means it when she says to "expect the unexpected." The series gives wide latitude to race directors to design each event to take best advantage of the course. And the race doesn't coddle participants by issuing a course map in advance of the race.

The Obstacles

Unlike some other obstacle races, Spartan doesn't let you skip obstacles without paying a price. And the legal tender in Sparta is burpees—10 to 30 per obstacle that you skip. Furthermore, you are strongly encouraged to at least try to overcome the obstacle before giving up and doing the burpees instead.

Spartan doesn't reveal in advance what obstacles any particular race features, but they do have the following staples in their obstacle repertoire:

Leap of Faith: Leap over a flaming bale of hay

The Mud Pit: Cross a muddy trench

Mt. Impossible: Climb an 8-foot wall

Heroes Spear Throw: Throw a spear at a target

Dark Tunnel: Crawl through a mud-covered tunnel

The Fallen: Fend off Spartan warriors armed with padded "jousting" clubs

Enemies Trap: Climb a cargo net

Slippery Victory: Climb a greased up 12-foot slippery wall built at a 45-degree angle

Barbed Crawl: Crawl under barbed wire

Expert Advice

Carrie Adams, brand manager for Spartan Race and participant in multiple races, says that how far in advance you want to start training depends on how fit you want to be for the run. "Three months in advance, you'll be in really good shape. Two months, decent shape. Some people don't prepare at all and that's fine, too. You'll have more fun if you do, though."

Super Spartan

Super Spartan is a more challenging version of the Spartan Sprint, featuring a longer course and more difficult obstacles.

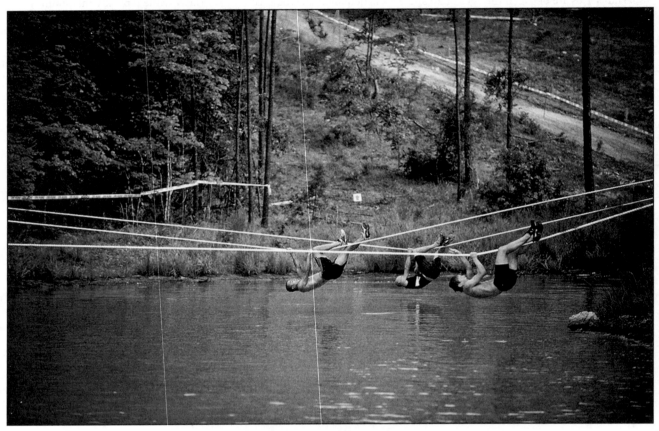

(Photo courtesy of Nuvision Action Image)

The Down and Dirty

Locations: A dozen events throughout the United States and Canada

Course: 8 or more miles

Level of Difficulty: Cringe and bear it

How Dirty Will You Get? Third-degree dirty

How Many Finish? 80 to 85 percent

Postrace Activities: Postrace festivities featuring DJs, food tents, and beer

Website: spartanrace.com/super-spartan-obstacle-course-race.html

Event Atmosphere

You won't find many costumes at this event, but you'll see a lot of well-chiseled eye candy—both male and female varieties. Participants are here to challenge themselves and to finish ahead of you.

What to Expect

To avoid backups and force the best out of you the first time, Spartan only gives you one attempt at its obstacles. If you fail, it's off to burpees hell for you. After a few sets of these cardio blasters, you'll be cursing yourself not training more seriously for this race.

The Obstacles

Spartan doesn't reveal in advance what obstacles any particular race features, but they do have the following staples in their obstacle repertoire:

Leap of Faith: Leap over a flaming bale of hay

The Mud Pit: Cross a muddy trench

Mt. Impossible: Climb an 8-foot wall

Heroes Spear Throw: Throw a spear at a target

Dark Tunnel: Crawl through a mud covered tunnel

The Fallen: Fend off Spartan warriors armed with padded "jousting" clubs

Enemies Trap: Climb a cargo net

Slippery Victory: Climb a greased up 12-foot slippery wall built at a 45-degree angle

Barbed Crawl: Crawl under barbed wire

Expert Advice

This race features long, challenging runs between obstacles, so if you don't want to suffer (or walk), make sure that you can run long distances over hilly and rough terrain.

Superhero Scramble

As if mud, ice-cold water, and flaming obstacles aren't enough, the folks behind the Superhero Scramble introduced a novel feature to their obstacle race course menu: Super Slime, a slick green ooze they use to coat the surfaces of several of their obstacles.

Various waves include a team and individual component, a singles wave, and the competitive Scramble Gamble wave.

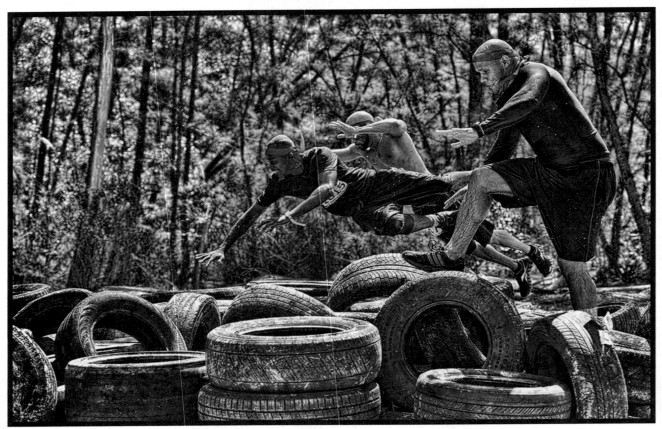

(Photo courtesy of the Superhero Scramble)

The Down and Dirty

Locations: Deerfield Beach (north Florida) and Miami, FL

Course: 4- to 6-mile course peppered with more than 20 obstacles

Level of Difficulty: Couch potatoes welcome!

How Dirty Will You Get? Third-degree dirty

How Many Finish? 95 percent

Postrace Activities: Postrace party featuring food trucks, live music, and beer

Website: superheroscramble.com

Event Atmosphere

An intimate race in which most participants dress as their favorite superheroes or wear last year's Halloween costumes. Treat this as a day to act like a kid again.

What to Expect

Expect more water crossings than at many other events, including a brief swim. Additionally, long lines are common, so if you're not into catching a breather, swapping war stories with fellow queue members, and taking pictures of your friends, plan to reach the obstacles before everyone else or skip this race.

The Obstacles

Superhero Scramble claims to have the most obstacle-dense courses, featuring a minimum of 20 obstacles. If you fail to complete an obstacle, you have to do Super Spins (10 spins with your forehead on a pole).

Here's what you can expect to encounter:

Wall Climbs: Hoist yourself up and over walls of varying heights

Water Crossings: Slog, swim, and slurp your way through watery obstacles

Marine Mile Bootcamp: Perform burpees, bear walks, and army crawls

Fire Jumps: Leap over flaming obstacles

Barbed Wire Mud Crawls: Slither under low-slung barbed wire without getting snagged

Balance Beams: Stay upright while maneuvering across a narrow beam or log

Rope Swings: Grab a rope and hang on for the ride

Ice-Cold Water: Plunge into a frigid pit

Slime Slide: Shoot down a slimed-up slide

Slip N' Slime: Try not to slip in the slime

Expert Advice

Wear a costume. It sets the mood and tone for a fun and adventurous day.

The Survival Race

Calling all couch potatoes! This one's for you. Survival Race owner Dean Del Prete says that he read a news story about obstacle racing and thought, "Holy cow, this puts the fun in fitness." So he proceeded to install obstacle courses at his paintball businesses around the country. The races are designed to give beginners a taste of what obstacle course racing is all about without all the adrenaline and intensity involved in many other events.

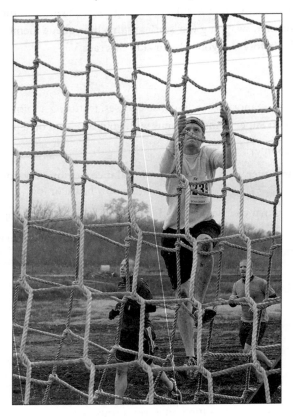

(Photo courtesy of the Survival Race)

The Down and Dirty

Locations: Dallas, TX; New Windsor, NY; Manchester, NJ; Long Island, NY; Toledo, OH (and coming soon to Virginia, North Carolina, and Florida)

Course: 5k course featuring 12 to 14 general obstacles per racecourse and 4 to 6 additional site-specific obstacles

Level of Difficulty: Couch potatoes welcome!

How Dirty Will You Get? Third-degree dirty

How Many Finish? 99 percent

Postrace Activities: Don't expect much of a postrace party, but there is a live band or DJ, and food/beverage vendors may or may not be available

Website: survivalrace.com

Event Atmosphere

A family-friendly atmosphere in which kids as young as 9 years old are encouraged to participate. Kids too young to enter the race can play on mini obstacles and join in on other activities. The goal of these races is to get people out moving and have fun doing it.

What to Expect

Obstacles aren't as challenging as in many other races, and almost everyone who starts the race finishes it. But do plan on getting very dirty, as the race says that it's "survival of the filthiest" rather than "survival of the fittest."

The Obstacles

Obstacles vary from course to course, but here are some of the usual suspects:

Loch Ness: You might have to swim through parts of this watery obstacle

Black Widow Cargo Net: Clamber up and over this 25-foot-tall obstacle strung with cargo netting

Black Beard's Plank: Put one foot in front of the other on a narrow log crossing over a creek or other water obstacle

Survival Sludge: Slog through a muddy pit

Tires of Terror: Step through a series of tires

Barbed Wire Belly Bopper: Avoid getting snagged on low-slung barbed wire as you make your way through a mud pit

Pipe Dream Crawl: Crawl through tunnels made with camouflage netting

Mt. Mud: Climb up a muddy hill

Fire Frenzy: Leap over a small pile of flaming logs

Expert Advice

No training necessary. Get off your butt and move … and bring the kids along, too!

Tough Mudder

The whole basis of Tough Mudder is that it's not a race, it's a challenge, with obstacles based on military training. And like its military inspiration, Mudder places a heavy emphasis on teamwork. Participants aren't timed because the goal is to finish, not win. That being said, Mudder does have a serious competitive component: if you finish in the top 5 percent of your event, you qualify for the World's Toughest Mudder, an annual 24-hour-long event with a $10,000 cash prize.

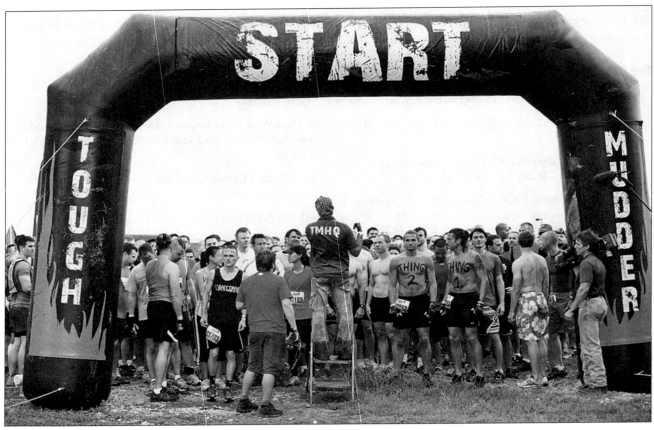

(Dmitry Gudkov for Tough Mudder)

The Down and Dirty

Locations: Courses across the United States, United Kingdom, Australia, and Canada. Venues may vary from year to year, but the same regions are always represented and all courses are within a couple hours of major metropolitan areas.

Course: 10 to 12 miles and 25 to 30 obstacles

Level of Difficulty: Cringe and bear it

How Dirty Will You Get? Third-degree dirty

How Many Finish? 80 percent

Postrace Activities: Dos Equis postparty with burgers and beer

Website: toughmudder.com

Event Atmosphere

You'll notice that the *R* word doesn't apply here: *Race*. Tough Mudder isn't an opportunity to *beat* anyone. It's not a test of how much time you can spend training or how many trees you can fell with your teeth. The events are personal challenges with the goal being simply to finish the course. Participants aren't timed and are encouraged to help one another dominate the obstacles—because nothing says "I love you" quite like hoisting a friend over a lubed-up half-pipe.

And as intense as the courses are, Mudders are ultimately looking for a good time. Teams compete in a variety of ridiculous costumes, and it's hard to be all Arnold circa 1984 when you're covered in mud and up against an obstacle called "Just the Tip." About equal parts men and women take part in Tough Mudder events. At the end of the day, it's all about having fun, sharing a beer, and finding the perfect place for your Tough Mudder tattoo.

Note: Spectators must purchase tickets to watch the race and attend the postrace party. Spectators tickets are pricy—$40 in 2012—but are discounted 50 percent if purchased in advance online.

What to Expect

Participants aren't timed because the goal is to finish, not win; teamwork is encouraged; must pledge to help fellow athletes and not whine.

The Obstacles

Tough Mudder has some of the most psychologically challenging obstacles in the business. There's no rule against skipping obstacles, but even foregoing a morning dose of Electroshock Therapy leaves you with a grueling course. And while each course is tailor-made for your very own excruciation, some of the classic obstacles include:

Greased Lightning: Slide down a steep hill into the pond and swim back out

Arctic Enema: Climb into and out of one of multiple lined dumpsters containing icy water and colored dye

Ball Shrinker: Traverse ropes stretched across a pond

Twinkle Toes: Walk across a narrow board over a river or pond

Devil's Beard: Crawl through low cargo nets

Nature's Pocket: Descend into 25 feet of underground tunnels

Electroshock Therapy: Run through a field of live electric wires, some of which deliver a 10,000-volt jolt

Everest: Scale a steep, slick quarter pipe structure covered in oil

Expert Advice

You need to be in good condition to man—or woman—handle these obstacles, so complete slackers need not apply. The minimum recommendation is that you're running regularly (two-plus times a week, working up to 5 miles per run), able to do 15 to 25 push-ups in a row, can bang out 6 pull-ups in a row (especially the dudes), and able to swim 50 yards without stopping (although you can skip the water obstacles). But while running regularly is part of the training regimen, a large share of Mudders have never run 10 miles straight before. It's not necessary to be a marathoner or half-marathoner, as the drudgery of running in a straight line is broken up with treats like belly-crawling, wall-climbing, mud-slogging, log-slinging, ice-water dunking, and enormous slip n' slides.

Warrior Dash

The Warrior Dash is a well-organized race series that is a great event for first-timers and is particularly popular among women runners. The world's largest running series is held on 65 challenging and rugged terrains across the world. Participants bound over fire, trudge through mud, and scale over 14 obstacles during this fierce 5k. After pushing their limits and conquering extreme obstacles, warriors celebrate with live music, grub, and beer.

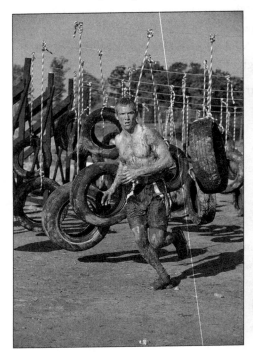 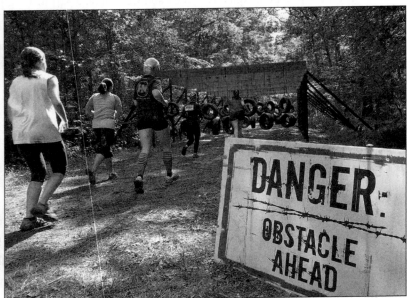

(Photos courtesy of Red Frog Events)

The Down and Dirty

Locations: 65 events around the world

Course: 5k (3.2 miles) featuring at least 14 obstacles

Level of Difficulty: Couch potatoes welcome!

How Dirty Will You Get? Third-degree dirty

How Many Finish? 98 percent

Postrace Activities: Beer tent with live music and food

Website: warriordash.com

Event Atmosphere

A participant described the Warrior Dash as a "5k party," and I think that does a pretty good job of summing up the atmosphere at this event. This is an all-day party with thousands of warriors hanging out before and after the race.

What to Expect

Don't expect a highly competitive event; this one is more for people of any fitness level who want to enjoy the course. Difficulty levels vary by location, with the most challenging races involving high elevations with steep hills to overcome, such as Copper Mountain, Colorado, or Windham Mountain, New York.

The Obstacles

Warrior Dash's obstacles are fairly straightforward and relatively easy to overcome:

Tornado Alley: Expect gale-force winds at the start of the race

Tunnels of Terror: Push through the pipe crawl

Deadweight Drifter: Slog through waist-deep water clogged with drifting logs

Hell's Hill: Sprint up to the top of a hill

Junkyard Jump: Make your way through a scrap yard

Walk the Plank: Put one foot in front of the other—it's exactly what it sounds like

Knee High Hill: Step through hundreds of tires

Great Warrior Wall: Climb a wooden barricade

Hay Fever: Climb over huge hay bales

Rio Run: Sprint down river

Cliffhanger: Rappel down a ravine

Cargo Climb: Go up and over a cargo net

Warrior Roast: Leap the flames

Muddy Mayhem: Crawl under barbed wire

Expert Advice

Bottlenecks are common at the obstacles, so it's a good idea to get out ahead of the pack in the early part of the race. However, a drawback to this tactic is that if you're not in shape, you're going to lose steam midway through the course.

Chapter 3

The Obstacles

Mud. Freezing water. Flames. Walls. Zombies. Expect any and all of the above out on the course. Although the exact obstacles change from event to event and year to year, they all tend to have clever names designed to play off your fears. Names like Electroshock Therapy, Petrifying Plunge, and Wall of Terror pretty much say it all.

Oh yeah—and they all claim to have been designed by Navy SEALS, British Special Forces, and other specialists in the art of "tough."

So a tough challenge requires a tough, careful approach. Renowned competitor Hobie Call offers this advice: "The last thing I want to do is injure myself on an obstacle and ruin my race, or possibly multiple races. So I tend to approach the obstacles carefully and methodically," he said. "Going through obstacles with acrobatic moves rarely helps, and just increases the odds of getting hurt."

This chapter provides a detailed breakdown of each race's challenges and obstacles, along with strategies to prepare you to conquer each.

Our Team of Experts

If you were to ask a group of obstacle racers to name their favorite and least favorite obstacles, you would find that their answers vary widely, and usually map pretty closely to each individual's strengths and weaknesses. People who don't have a lot of upper-body strength prefer the obstacles that require leg strength rather than arm strength, while those with good grip strength and Popeyelike pipes tend to have warm and fuzzy feelings for the monkey bars, rope climbs, and haul and carries. Similarly, competitors who are blessed with good balance often list obstacles—such as the log hop and balance beam—that require equilibrium under difficult conditions among their favorites. And it should go without saying that our pet neuroses have a significant influence on our attitudes toward obstacles: claustrophobics dislike tunnels and chutes, poor swimmers abhor the water obstacles, and people with a fear of heights get woozy when thinking about cargo net climbs.

Your strengths and weaknesses—not to mention your fears and anxieties—play a big part in determining the best strategy for approaching each obstacle. Because people have varied skill sets, there is no one-size-fits-all approach for attacking the obstacles. That's why I've assembled a team of experts with a wide range of skills and athletic backgrounds, and asked them to share their favorite approaches for tackling the many obstacles you'll encounter.

Hobie Call: The world's premier obstacle racer, Hobie has won six Spartan races in a row, and also holds the world record for the fastest lunging mile.

Tip

Hobie reminds racers that obstacles are only part of the race, so you shouldn't push yourself any harder than you do when you're running. "You want to pace yourself through the obstacles just like you do between them," he advises.

Carrie Adams: Carrie is founder and CEO of Rad Racing (radracing.org), a company committed to providing brand management, promotion, and consulting for traditional and nontraditional endurance races and challenges worldwide. She founded Spartan Chicked, a female-friendly movement engaging thousands of women across the globe to seek out a healthier way of living, training, and racing beyond the pavement.

Amelia Boone: Amelia has been hooked on obstacle and adventure racing ever since tackling Tough Mudders, Spartan races, and the GORUCK and SERE challenges. She is the female winner of the 2012 Winter Death Race, a race lasting for over 32 hours, and took second place for women at the inaugural 2011 World's Toughest Mudder 24-hour race.

Joe Decker: A two-time Spartan Death Race winner, Joe is recognized as "The World's Fittest Man." He is an ultra-endurance power athlete, renowned Boot Camp instructor, and motivational speaker who has helped thousands of women and men take control of their lives, realizing their true fitness potential.

Junyong Pak: He has won the inaugural 2011 World's Toughest Mudder 24-hour race and has been a top three finisher in numerous other Spartan races and Tough Mudders, including a third place finish at the 2011 Spartan World Championship.

Margaret Schlachter: Margaret's blog, dirtinyourskirt.com, won the Best Sports Blog award at the 2012 Weblog Awards. Her objective is to be the best-known female obstacle racer as well as a top competitor in endurance races.

Stew Smith, CSCS: A graduate of the U.S. Naval Academy, a former Navy SEAL Lieutenant, and author of several fitness and self-defense books. Stew has trained thousands of students for Navy SEALs, Special Forces, SWAT, FBI, ERT, and many other military and law enforcement professions.

Tip

Jane Di Leo of Tough Mudder shared some of the more creative approaches people have taken to getting past TM's obstacles, which are designed to require teamwork.

For obstacles like Everest, which is a greasy quarter pipe to ascend, teams often station people at the top to catch the hands of those running up it, or build a human pyramid on top of the pipe. On the 14-foot Berlin Wall, people climb on a teammate's shoulders or squat down to make a basket out of their hands to hoist people up by their feet. "And honestly, some of it is just pacing each other, literally pushing or pulling each other through obstacles like the Boa Constrictor," she said.

Balance Beam

Traverse a narrow beam or log, often spanning a mud pit or water hazard.

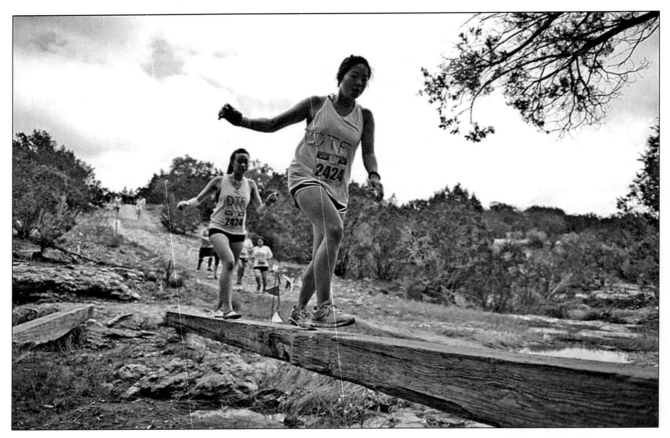

Muddy Buddies make their way across the balance beam.

(Photo courtesy of Muddy Buddy)

Expert Advice

Take stock of the situation before hopping on, advises Amelia. "If there are multiple people on the beam, wait until they get off as it will reduce the shaking. Move quickly across the beam, and keep your eyes fixed a few feet in front of you rather than straight down at your feet." If you're having trouble maintaining your balance, Boone suggests switching to Plan B: "If you're very unsteady and the rules allow it, scoot across on your bottom."

Once you're on the beam, Margaret says to "Take one step at a time and use your arms for balance."

Joe warns against spending too much time on this obstacle: "Line up, get your head straight, and haul ass. If you fall it's generally into mud or water and sometimes faster."

Note

The most challenging obstacles are the ones that require balance, according to Junyong: "My balance is good, but I think when you combine a need for balance with lack of breath, and then add a psychological aspect to it—you're chasing somebody or getting chased—it's so much easier to fail. In normal practice, it's super simple because your mind is relaxed. But when you *have* to make it across, that's when you tend to fail. That's where I have the most trouble."

How does Pak train to get better at handling the added pressure of remaining balanced during a race? Practice: "I've re-created the zigzag beam in my backyard, and figured out a technique that gets me across every time even if out of breath or in panic."

Obstacle-Specific Training Exercises

Target Muscle Groups	Suggested Exercises
Primary	
Legs	Lunges, squats, standing calf raises
Core	Planks, torso rotations
Secondary	
Shoulders	Dumbbell lateral raises

Cargo Net Climb

Clamber up a cargo net to the top of an obstacle. Once you reach the top, you either have to jump or climb the net down to the other side.

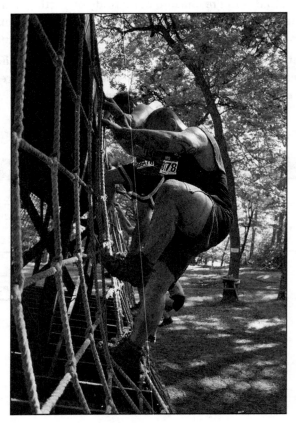

Participants competing on the Cargo Climb in the Warrior Dash.

(Photo courtesy of Red Frog Events)

Expert Advice

The best way to attack this obstacle is to climb facing the net rather than putting your back to it. Use your arms to pull and your legs to push, place your feet securely on the rope, and grasp the rope with both hands.

Obstacle-Specific Training Exercises

Target Muscle Groups	Suggested Exercises
Primary	
Legs	Squats, lunges, step-ups
Back	Pull-ups, pull-downs, dumbbell rows
Heart/lungs	Cardio intervals, running
Secondary	
Calves	Standing calf raises
Biceps	Chin-ups or chin-downs
Core	Torso rotations, planks, Superman back extensions
Forearms	Flexion and extension wrist curls
Hands and fingers	Finger flexion exercises such as tennis ball squeezes and grip master squeezes
Serratus anterior	Straight arm pullovers
Trapezius	Shoulder shrugs

Carry and Haul

Channel your inner pack animal as you lug heavy loads—logs, 5-gallon buckets filled with sand, sandbags, tires, and chunks of cement—from one point to another.

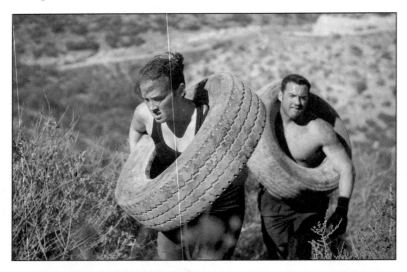

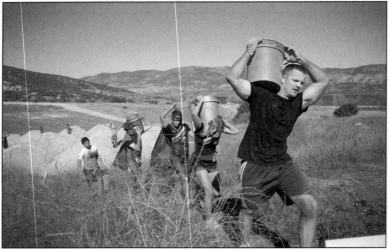

Spartan competitors haul heavy loads.

(Photos courtesy of Nuvision Action Image)

Race directors like to get sadistic with the carry by combining it with other challenges. You might have to haul your booty up steep, sandy hills, through waist deep water, or through other obstacles, such as hay bale mounds or tires. GORUCK's variation on this challenge is a group carry, which poses its own set of unique trials requiring tremendous patience and teamwork.

Expert Advice

For particularly heavy or cumbersome objects, Junyong cautions against running. Instead, he suggests "walking slowly and steadily. Change holding positions frequently to give your muscles a break."

Hobie chimes in with advice for staying safe during this challenge: "When carrying sandbags, tires, or logs on a hillside, hold them on the side of your body that is away from the hill. That way if you slip, you can use your free hand to catch yourself. This is a good way to avoid injury and keep moving quicker."

And Stew offers his perspective as a trainer: "Make sure to train your core muscles to handle being off balance while carrying heavy objects."

Note

Your hands, forearms, and shoulders are often the first to tire when hauling heavy objects. You can give yourself an edge over other competitors by strengthening the muscles in these areas.

Obstacle-Specific Training Exercises

Target Muscle Groups	Suggested Exercises
Primary	
Back	Deadlifts; barbell, dumbbell, or machine rows; back flies
Arms, forearms, and hands	Biceps curls; forearm flexion and extension wrist curls; finger flexion exercises such as hang from an overhead bar, tennis ball squeezes, and grip master squeezes
Shoulders	Shoulder presses, front raises, lateral raises, reverse flies, shoulder shrugs (traps)
Secondary	
Legs	Squats, lunges, step-ups, standing calf raises
Core	Planks, torso rotations, knee/leg raises

Crawls—Under

Snake your way under low-lying objects, such as barbed wire or netting. Many obstacles include a mud feature in their crawls, putting you face-first in the sloppy mix. When race designers are feeling particularly sadistic, they install crawls up steep hills, forcing you to slither against gravity.

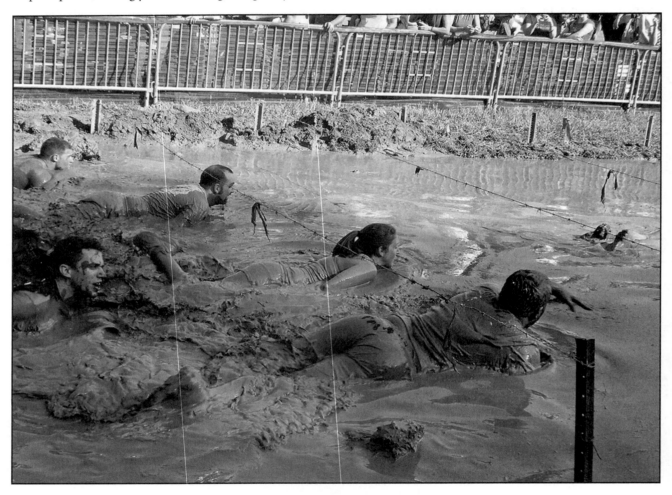

Warriors get down and dirty to avoid the barbed wire.

(Photo courtesy of Red Frog Events)

Expert Advice

Most people army crawl by lying on their stomachs and moving forward using the arm and leg on the same side of the body together. But Hobie has perfected a much faster strategy: rolling under the obstacles. You can go faster and expend less energy. Log rolling isn't always possible, though, particularly when you have to go uphill, the course zigzags, or if the barbed wire is hung too low.

Another favorite strategy for kicking the snot out of the barbed wire obstacle is to take a standard plank position and plank your way all the way through. You essentially pull yourself forward using those forearms and press off the toes as you thrust forward. Not only will you soar through while others just manage, but you will save your knees from the typical cuts and bruises. This technique requires lots of upper-body strength, especially in the back and shoulders.

Obstacle Ahead!

Dr. Michael Camp advises athletes to "avoid the barbed wire or electric fence obstacles if your back already feels stiff or uncomfortable. If you try to compensate for the discomfort while going through the obstacle, you can either make the injury worse or hurt another part of your body."

Obstacle-Specific Training Exercises

Target Muscle Groups	Suggested Exercises
Primary	
Legs	Squats, lunges, deadlifts, hip extensions, standing calf raises
Core	Planks, bicycle maneuvers, torso rotations, Superman back extensions
Secondary	
Back	Straight arm pullovers, dumbbell rows

Log Hop

Jump from stump to stump without losing your balance.

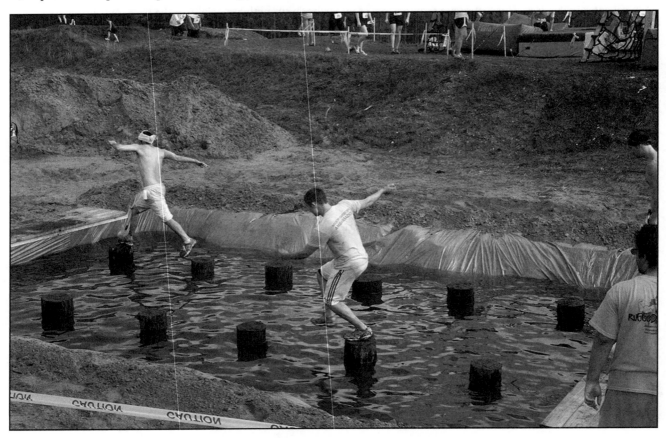

Try not to get stumped by the log hop at the Rugged Maniac.

(Photo courtesy of Rugged Races LLC)

Some courses place the stumps in water; others fill the obstacle with mud, making you pay a dirty price if you lose your balance.

Expert Advice

According to Amelia, the trick to conquering this obstacle is to "sink low into a squat and leap using your legs if you have a distance to cover. Take your time to regain your balance before you leap again."

Margaret likes to pause and study the obstacle for a moment to try to find the best line for getting through it. And if you really want to own this obstacle? Schlachter says that you should practice at home on logs set at low heights.

Junyong advises to take a couple of deep breaths before attacking the log hop. You'll need that extra breath because, "just when you think you've got it, oftentimes there's a spin. Like at the Spartan championship race, usually I get to an obstacle first so it's squeaky clean, but during championship they had us go last so it was all muddy and some of the logs were uneven. There's no particularly good way to approach it except to have a very cool head about it."

Obstacle Ahead!

"Some of the logs are less secure, and that can throw off your balance," warns Carrie. "As you jump from log to log, be mindful that it might not be a firm landing."

Obstacle-Specific Training Exercises

Target Muscle Groups	Suggested Exercises
Primary	
Legs	Squats, squat jumps, box jumps, lunge jumps, leg extensions, leg curls, standing calf raises
Secondary	
Core	Planks, torso rotations, bicycle maneuvers

Over-Under-Through

Climb over and under and through a maze of ladder walls or other obstacles. The watery version of this obstacle involves floating logs or other objects that you must swim or duck under and climb over.

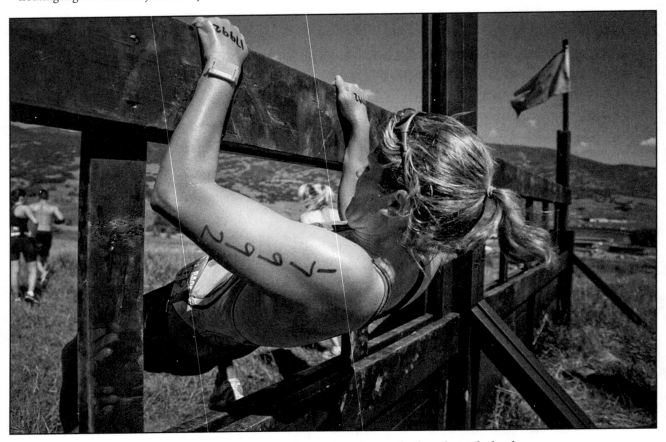

This Spartan competitor makes going through the obstacle look easy.

(Photo courtesy of Nuvision Action Image)

Expert Advice

Amelia Boone likes to survey the terrain as she approaches this obstacle so that she can map out a route. "Look for the lower parts to hop over, and the higher clearances to go under," she recommends, adding, "take note of any mud or hazards that you want to avoid."

Use both your arms and legs to get through the obstacle. Don't rush the walls. You will need to be flexible and use your whole body.

Obstacle-Specific Training Exercises

Target Muscle Groups	Suggested Exercises
Primary	
Legs	Squats, lunges, calf raises
Back	Pull-ups or pull-downs, dumbbell rows, dumbbell or straight arm pullovers
Arms	Chin-ups, biceps curls
Secondary	
Heart/lungs	Cardio intervals, running, swimming

Pipe/Chute Crawl

Crawl through a tunnel or pipe. Tunnels might be underground, through the water, or through the mud.

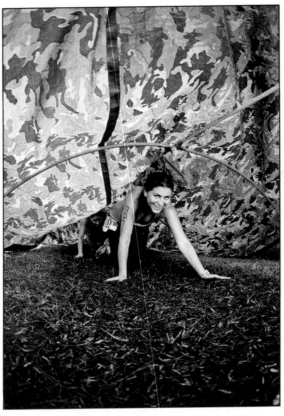

Get as low to the ground as possible in the chute crawl.

(Photo courtesy of Run For Your Lives)

Expert Advice

To make an obstacle like this as effortless as possible, you want your upper- and lower-body muscles to work in concert with each other. As you use your legs to push off of the ground, use your arms to reach and pull, or keep your arms close in and push off using your forearms. Getting your muscles to work together helps conserve energy and gets you through without burning out any one muscle group.

Hobie adds: "Stay low to the ground and be sure to breathe properly. Use small movements because the space is tight."

Obstacle-Specific Training Exercises

Target Muscle Groups	Suggested Exercises
Primary	
Legs	Squats, lunges, deadlifts, hip extensions, standing calf raises
Core	Planks, bicycle maneuvers, torso rotations, Superman back extensions
Secondary	
Back	Straight arm pullovers, dumbbell rows
Shoulders	Any bench press movement with a front shoulder raise

Fire Leap

Leap over a fire made of burning logs or hay bales.

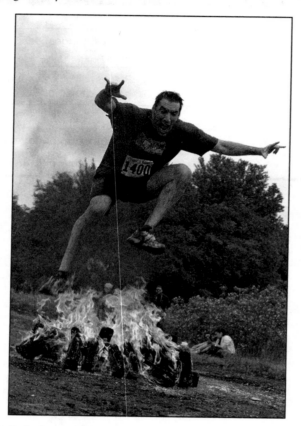

A Rebel Racer leaps over a flaming obstacle.

(Photo courtesy of Oz Sports Photography)

Expert Advice

Step up to the obstacle and make sure that you have good footing. Look over the obstacle and identify a level, dry landing spot. Take an aggressive, well-timed jump toward your landing spot.

Obstacle Ahead!

For safety reasons, races keep this obstacle fairly simple—but you should use extreme caution. Keep in mind that what might seem like a short distance at the beginning of the race can feel like a gaping void when you're exhausted.

Obstacle-Specific Training Exercises

Target Muscle Groups	Suggested Exercises
Primary	
Legs	Long jump, squats, squat jumps, box jumps, lunge jumps, leg extensions, leg curls, standing calf raises
Secondary	
Heart/lungs	Running, cardio intervals
Core	Planks, torso rotations, bicycle maneuvers

Hill Climbs

Run up and down hills of various length and steepness. Climbs can involve very tricky footing, deep sand, boulders, and other objects that make footing very difficult.

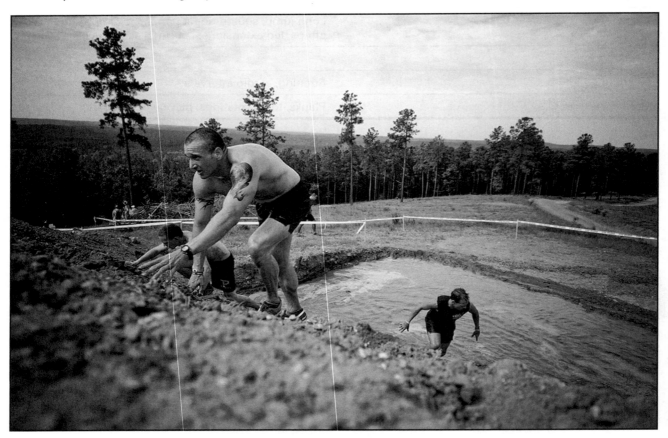

Pace yourself on the hill climbs at the Super Spartan.

(Photo courtesy of Nuvision Action Image)

Expert Advice

When you're up against a steep mountain, you'll wish you had trained for such a challenge. Remember, you're already beat up from having conquered other obstacles … and now this! This is an obstacle where you often see racers stopped, trying to allow their exhausted leg muscles to recover and/or their tapped-out lungs and cardio to rekindle.

When going uphill, sprint for a distance, then stop and recover. It allows you to cover more ground, faster. Yes, you can certainly try to run up the mountain in one shot, but you'll likely burn out before you get there—to the point of not being able to recover—risking a groin muscle or hamstring pull. Instead, pace yourself and sprint in 15- to 20-second bursts, resting just long enough to catch your breath.

Joe suggests your plan of attack for hills should depend on the length of the race: "In a 5k lean forward and pump like hell to get up it and keep going. In a longer event, take your time, lean into the hill, and power walk up it." And if you're in a grueling event such as the Spartan Beast or the World's Toughest Mudder, Decker offers up this bit of gallows humor: "On day two just lie down face first and crawl to the top."

General running techniques can make a big difference on hills, too. When running up hills, keep your body low to the ground, take smaller steps, and explode off of each step. When running down hills, again use smaller steps to ensure balance is maintained.

Tip

Founder Amit Nar shared some tips for conquering the Rebel Race's Himalayas, a series of hills culminating in a slimy downward slide. "On the Himalayas, people can't get up the first hill; they keep sliding back down. You have to have some people at the top extending their hands, but then people at the top are in mud and they slide down. They land in the mud, it's like quicksand—once you get in, you can't get out. It honestly smells like poop. You have to help each other. It's a team effort, basically."

Obstacle-Specific Training Exercises

Target Muscle Groups	Suggested Exercises
Primary	
Legs	Lunges (especially pushing off of the toes, which will ignite those quads!), weighted step-ups, squats
Heart/lungs	Running, cardio intervals
Secondary	
Shoulders/core	Planks
Back	Dumbbell, barbell, or machine rows; neutral-grip pull-ups or pull-downs

Hurdles

Climb or jump over hurdles of various heights.

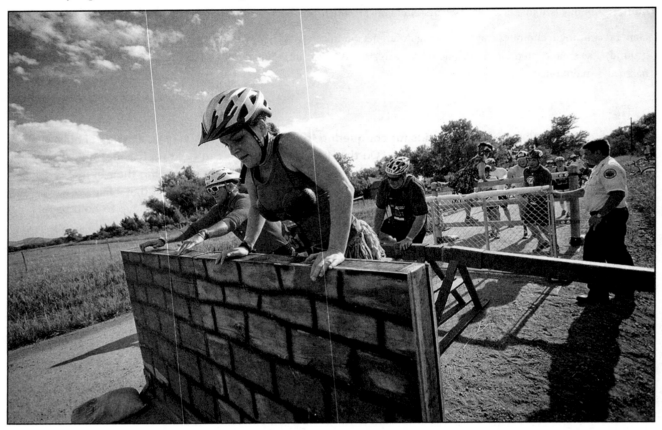

Muddy Buddies attack a series of hurdles.

(Photo courtesy of Muddy Buddy)

Expert Advice

"Unless you were a college track star," Amelia advises, "place your hands to one side of the hurdle and hop over." To really get the most lift, Margaret recommends jumping with your feet at the same time that you press down with your arms. And Joe says to attack the hurdles aggressively and push off forcefully with your legs.

Obstacle-Specific Training Exercises

Target Muscle Groups	Suggested Exercises
Primary	
Legs	Squat jumps, lunge jumps, box jumps, squats, lunges, calf raises
Triceps	Triceps dips
Shoulders	Shoulder presses, front shoulder raises, dumbbell lateral raises
Secondary	
Core	Reverse crunches, leg/knee raises

Incline Wall

Climb an inclined wall using a rope or hand grips. To make this obstacle more challenging, some races coat the surface of the wall with water, grease, or slime, making it even more difficult to keep your footing.

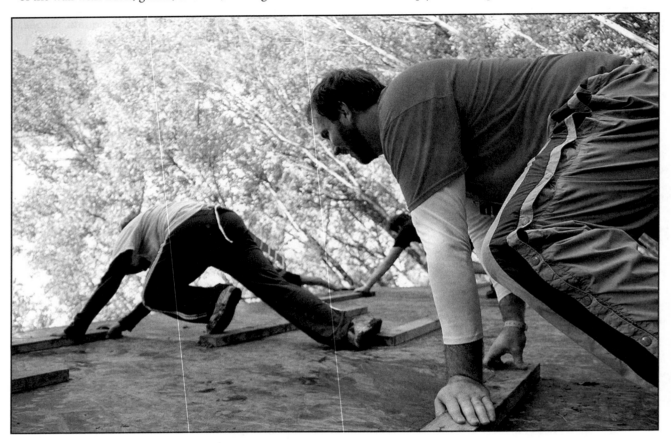

Scaling the incline wall at Run For Your Lives.

(Photo courtesy of Run For Your Lives)

Expert Advice

Hand grip is the key to this obstacle. Before putting any weight on the rope, make sure that you have a good hold on it. Amelia recommends wearing a pair of grippy gloves for extra hold, and also to protect your hands.

Once you have a good grip, place your feet wide apart and flat against the surface to help maintain balance. If the surface is greased, push straight down into the wall with your feet (rather than pushing back) to maintain your balance and propel yourself forward and upward.

Tip

Junyong notes that races often have obstacles requiring grip strength right after a mud or water obstacle, which makes the grips incredibly slippery. To practice, he recommends hanging off a pull-up bar with wet hands.

Obstacle-Specific Training Exercises

Target Muscle Groups	Suggested Exercises
Primary	
Hands and fingers	Finger flexion exercises such as tennis ball squeezes and grip master squeezes
Serratus anterior	Straight arm pullovers
Trapezius	Shoulder shrugs
Legs	Squats, lunges, step-ups
Secondary	
Back	Pull-ups, pull-downs, dumbbell rows
Heart/lungs	Cardio intervals, running

Joust

Run through a gauntlet of beefy guys trying to club you with padded "jousting" sticks.

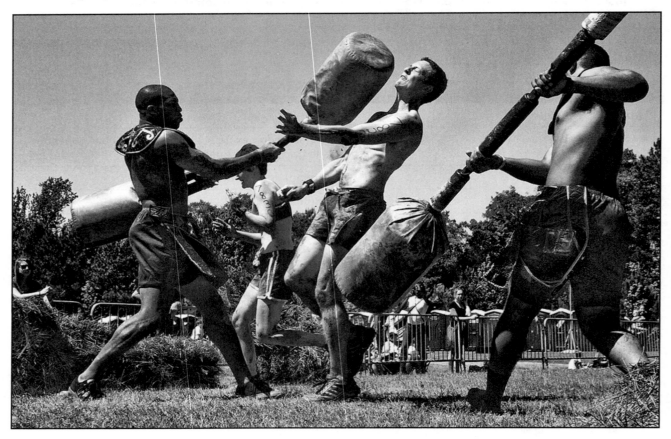

Competitors must overcome one final obstacle—the joust—before crossing the finish line at this Spartan race.

(Photo courtesy of Nuvision Action Image)

Expert Advice

Don't let these guys scare you, but also avoid engaging with them if you can. "And don't leave your feet!" advises Carrie. "The last thing you want is your legs swept out from underneath you at the end of a race."

Joe sums up the best way to attack this obstacle: "Put your shoulder down and run over them like Walter Payton!"

Obstacle-Specific Training Exercises

Target Muscle Groups	Suggested Exercises
Primary	
Legs	Speed drills, agility drills, squats, lunges, squat jumps, calf raises
Chest	Any chest pressing movements using dumbbells or barbells
Core	Bicycle maneuvers, planks, Swiss ball crunches
Secondary	
Arms	Close-grip bench presses using barbells or dumbbells, triceps dips, close-grip push-ups

Monkey Bars

Maneuver from bar to bar (or rope to rope) across the obstacle using your arms (or legs, if allowed). Race directors like to monkey around with this obstacle by greasing some or all of the bars, making them very difficult to grasp. Bars also often span water or a mud pit.

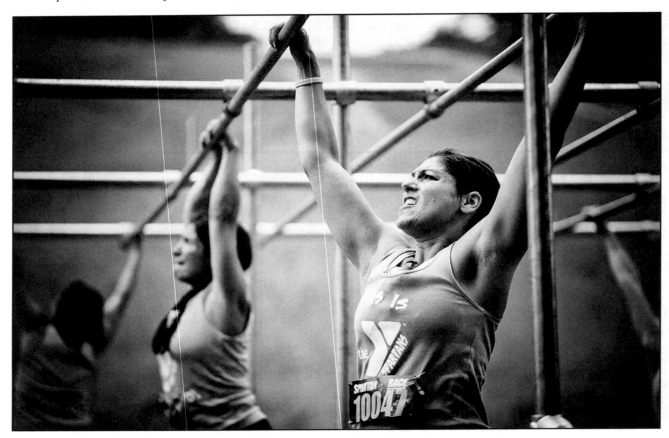

Monkey bars at a Spartan race in New York.

(Photo courtesy of Nuvision Action Image)

Expert Advice

You can have superhuman arm and shoulder strength, but if the monkey bars are slippery, you'll still struggle to get across. The swinging effect of your forward motion exacerbates slippages, so go slow, bend your arms at approximately 90 degrees, and use both hands at each bar. Try to keep your body from swaying too much. It's a choppier movement, and takes more overall energy, but your grip is much more secure this way. If you're comfortable wearing gloves, they can help you keep your grip, especially on cold days or if the bars are greased or wet.

Pak's solution to slippery monkey bars? Use your legs instead of your arms. Hang upside down from your ankles—or a combination of your ankles and hands—to reduce the load on your hands.

Tip

"Tough Mudder randomly greases some bars on its monkey bars, so you have to be careful," Hobie advises. "If the bars are dry and my hands are dry, I can skip a couple bars and get across in a couple seconds. If they are greased, if you start swinging you'll lose your grip, no matter how strong you are. So if the bars are slippery, you have to grab each bar with both hands and keep your body from swinging. I've had times when going across one like that I barely made it across. You have to be real careful about it."

Obstacle-Specific Training Exercises

Target Muscle Groups	Suggested Exercises
Primary	
Biceps/forearms	Chin-ups, direct gripping exercises such as hanging bar holds, tennis ball squeezes, and grip master squeezes
Hands and fingers	Finger flexion exercises such as tennis ball squeezes and grip master squeezes
Back	Pull-ups (either assisted, using full-body weight or added weight)
Shoulders	Shoulder presses, front shoulder raises, dumbbell lateral raises, reverse dumbbell shoulder flies
Secondary	
Core	Hanging knee/leg raises, planks, torso rotations, reverse crunches
Trapezius	Shoulder shrugs with dumbbells

Mud Pits

Walk or run through the knee- or even waist-deep mud.

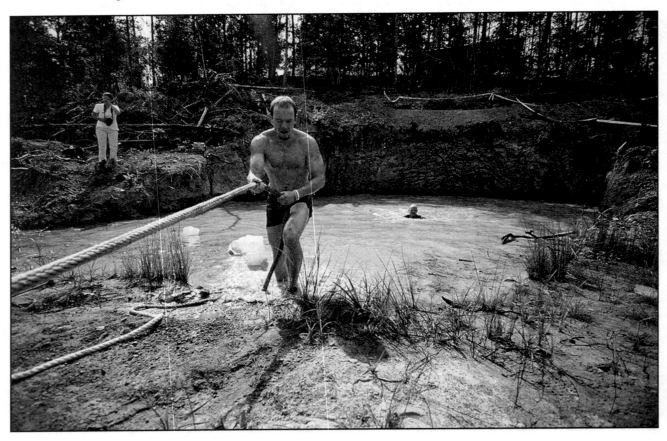

You need to grab a rope to extract yourself from some mud pits, such as the one at this Spartan race.

(Photo courtesy of Nuvision Action Image)

Expert Advice

Running through a mud pit might not only seem like an efficient mode of attack, but also a lot of fun. And it is—for about 30 seconds. After that, you'll be toast. Junyong says that the most efficient way to get through thick mud is by walking. "If you try to run you're burning so much more energy," he stresses. "You're going to be huffing and short of breath even if you're walking. Take long strides, pump your arms, and be careful of uneven footing."

Note

Mud pits are a great equalizer in obstacle races. Everyone's going to be going at the same pace.

Obstacle-Specific Training Exercises

Target Muscle Groups	Suggested Exercises
Primary	
Legs	Lunges, squats, step-ups, calf raises
Shoulders	Front raises, indirect work from all pressing movements
Secondary	
Core	Torso rotations, oblique crunches, reverse crunches
Third	
Heart/lungs	Cardio intervals, running

Tough Mudder's Everest Quarter-Pipe Climb

Scale a steep, greased quarter-pipe.

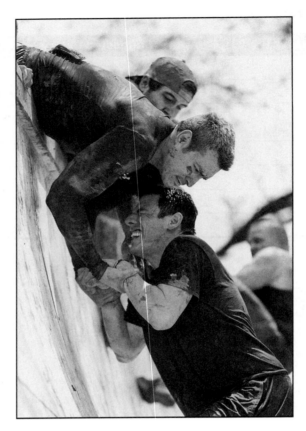

It takes teamwork to conquer Tough Mudder's Everest obstacle.

(Dmitry Gudkov for Tough Mudder)

The surface of the pipe is often coated in oil or some other slippery substance. And even if it wasn't intentionally made slick, it's often wet and muddy from the feet of runners who are ahead of you.

Expert Advice

Many participants rely on the goodwill of fellow competitors to lend them a helping hand up the pipe. To do it this way, get a good running start, propel yourself up the pipe as far as you can, and then reach up and try to grab the outstretched arms and hands of people waiting at the top, who then pull you the rest of the way up.

According to Junyong, going this one alone isn't easy, but it can be done. He shares his course-tested advice for scaling Everest solo: "Tough Mudder has quarter pipe—Everest—that seems completely impossible to do without help. When I encountered it for the third time, there was this manifold at the top covered with vegetable oil, which was super slippery. You fall flat on your face if you try to push off instead of deflecting off. But no matter how slippery a surface is, you can always push up from it."

Obstacle-Specific Training Exercises

Target Muscle Groups	Suggested Exercises
Primary	
Legs	Uphill sprints, squats, lunges, calf raises
Back	Dumbbell rows
Secondary	
Core	Oblique crunches, bicycle maneuvers, torso rotations

Rope Climb

Pull yourself up a rope. In most events the rope is knotted, giving you more purchase as you climb. Often there's a bell at the top that you must ring to signal the success of your ascent.

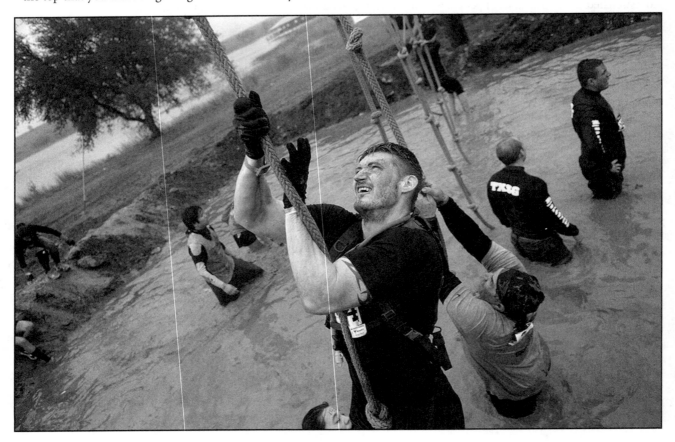

The rope climb at a Super Spartan in Texas requires a strong grip and steely determination.

(Photo courtesy of Nuvision Action Image)

Expert Advice

Grip strength is key here: keep your fingers clenched tightly around the rope.

Obstacle-Specific Training Exercises

Target Muscle Groups	Suggested Exercises
Primary	
Hands and fingers	Finger flexion exercises such as tennis ball squeezes and grip master squeezes
Forearms	Hammer curls, reverse curls, hanging rope holds, forearm flexion and extension wrist curls
Legs	Leg curls, adductor machine, wide stance squats, stiff leg deadlifts
Biceps	Chin-ups
Secondary	
Serratus anterior	Straight arm pullovers
Trapezius	Shoulder shrugs

Rope Traverse

Cross a single or double rope spanning a body of water.

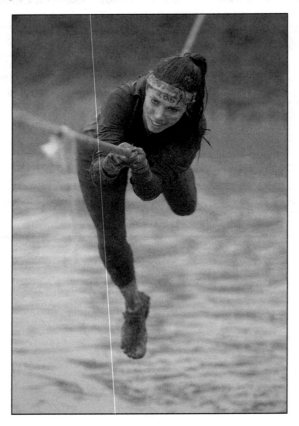

A Spartan competitor crosses a single rope spanning a river.

(Photo courtesy of Nuvision Action Image)

Expert Advice

Junyong suggests two strategies for this tricky obstacle, depending on the situation:

"Most people hang below the rope and drag their ankles and pull themselves like they're climbing a rope," says Junyong. "That's how I like to go, too, because it's faster," he adds. However, Tough Mudder often puts a plastic sheathe over the rope. In that case, Pak recommends getting wet (if you're not already), balancing yourself on top of the rope, and sliding across. "It's super efficient because you're only fighting friction, not gravity," he explains, "and being wet minimizes friction."

Obstacle-Specific Training Exercises

Target Muscle Groups	Suggested Exercises
Primary	
Legs	Wide stance squats, lunges, adductor machine, stiff leg deadlifts
Biceps and forearms	Chin-ups
Secondary	
Back	Neutral-grip rows

Sandy or Swampy Terrain

Obstacle race directors consider rough, difficult terrain of any sort to be fair game for their races. Expect to encounter thick sand, tree roots, deep ruts, rocks, and even swamps on the course.

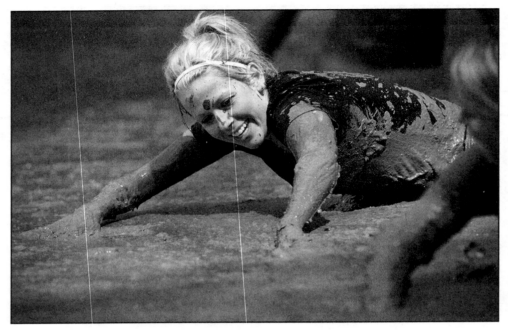

Expect to encounter rocky, muddy, or even swampy terrain in any obstacle race you enter.

(Photo courtesy of Nuvision Action Image)

Expert Advice

"Run to the edges or in trails already beaten down by those ahead of you," advises Amelia. "Watch out, though, as sometimes that can make it more slick. And make sure to tie your laces tight! I've known plenty of people to lose shoes in the mud or swamp."

Margaret says to raise your knees high, adding "The quicker you can move and the higher you can bring your feet up, the faster you will move through this challenging terrain. Don't stay in one place for more than a second, just keep moving at a consistent pace."

Obstacle-Specific Training Exercises

Target Muscle Groups	Suggested Exercises
Primary	
Legs	Squats, leg curls, stiff leg deadlifts
Secondary	
Shoulders	Front shoulder raises

Slides

Whiz down a large slide, often coated with mud or fed a constant supply of water. Slides usually dump riders into a mud or water pit.

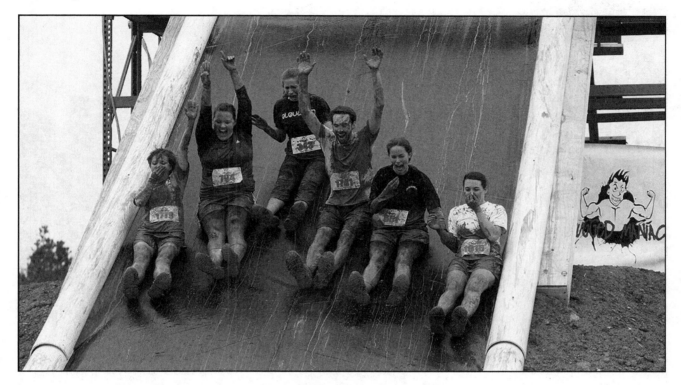

Rugged Maniac competitors plunge down a slide into a pool of water.

(Photo courtesy of Rugged Races LLC)

Expert Advice

There's really not much strategy involved in slides, besides hanging on and enjoying the ride. Take a deep breath and stay relaxed. Try to avoid getting mud splashed in your eyes when you land in the mud pit.

Obstacle Ahead!

Keep your core strong and your legs limp. If your legs are rigid and you hit the ground hard, you could sustain an ankle or knee injury.

Obstacle-Specific Training Exercises

Target Muscle Groups	Suggested Exercises
Core	Planks, torso rotations

Smoke

Run or walk through smoke.

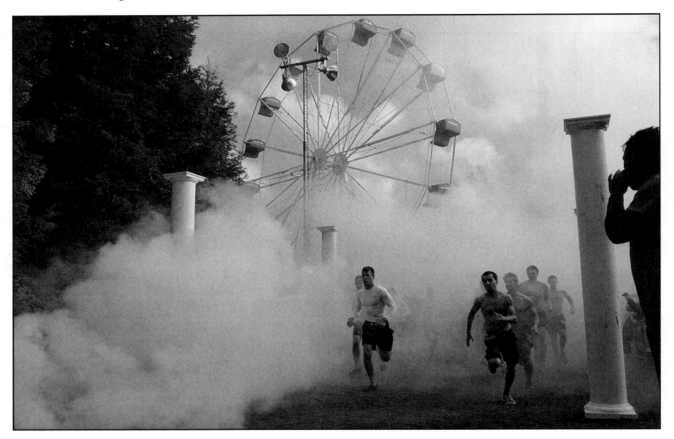

Smoke gets in the eyes of Spartan racers.

(Photo courtesy of Nuvision Action Image)

Expert Advice

All of our experts chimed in with variations on Joe's advice: "Run like hell!" Because you want to avoid breathing in any smoke, take a deep breath before encountering the smoke, and try to hold it until you get through it. Margaret suggests looking at the ground instead of ahead of you to help keep the smoke out of your eyes.

Obstacle-Specific Training Exercises

Target Muscle Groups	Suggested Exercises
Legs	Lunges, squats, calf raises
Heart/lungs	Sprinting or running

Tire Flips

Flip large tractor tires over and onto the other side.

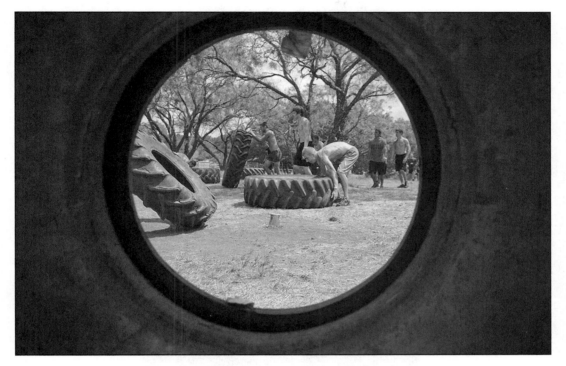

Spartan competitors tackle the tire flip.

(Photo courtesy of Nuvision Action Image)

Expert Advice

Joe recommends using a combination of grip strength and your legs to get underneath the tire. Next, do a deadlift, using your thigh strength to get the tire up onto its tread. Once you get it up, give it a shove and let gravity do the rest of the work. Oh, and one final piece of advice from Joe: "Attack the tire. Don't be a sissy."

The over/under grip that powerlifters often use with a barbell obviously won't work here, so take an underhand grip, but keep your arms tucked extremely tight into the sides of your body, so that your biceps are not actually lifting. The underhand grip functions as the forklift platform, while the legs and back muscles do the lifting.

Obstacle-Specific Training Exercises

Target Muscle Groups	Suggested Exercises
Legs	Squats, deep knee deadlifts
Shoulders	Push presses
Triceps	Close-grip bench presses

Tire Run

Run through a series of tires in this traditional military obstacle.

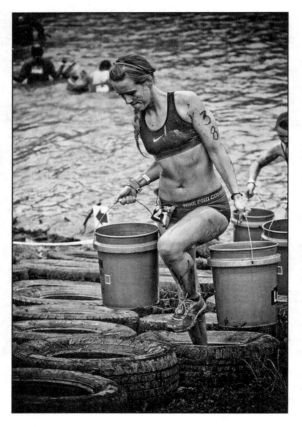

Spartan complicates the tire run by making competitors carry buckets of water.

(Photo courtesy of Nuvision Action Image)

Expert Advice

"Pump your arms and move your feet like Herschel Walker," commands Joe. Use quick, light movements and lift your knees high to get through each tire. Unlike balance events, where it's helpful to look a few feet in front of you rather than down at your feet, for tire runs you should watch where you step.

If you are light enough to stay on top of the tires, this is a good option for getting through the obstacle quickly.

Note

Margaret reports having had an out-of-body experience on a tire run at the World's Toughest Mudder. She was about 20 hours into the event when she encountered the tire run, and started to hallucinate. "I thought the blacktop below was water and the depths unknown, so I opted to walk on top of the tires."

Obstacle-Specific Training Exercises

Target Muscle Groups	Suggested Exercises
Primary	
Legs	Squats, leg curls, stiff leg deadlifts
Secondary	
Shoulders	Front shoulder raises

Throws—Spears or Rocks

Throw a spear or rock at a target.

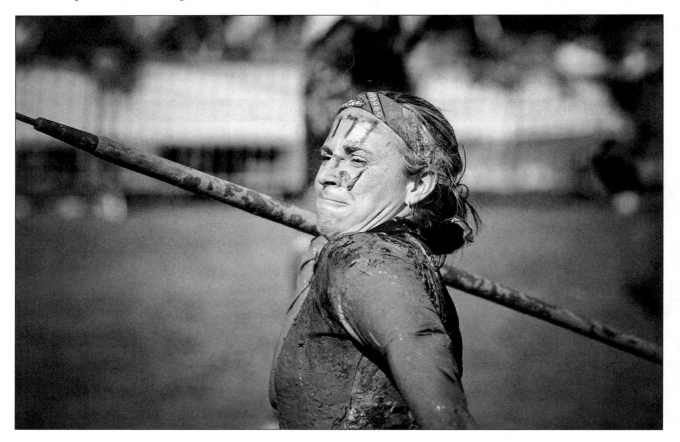

Channel your inner caveman during the spear throw.

(Photo courtesy of Nuvision Action Image)

Expert Advice

"Throwing a spear is different than throwing a baseball or football," says Amelia. "Remember that the butt of the spear is long, so you need to loft it like a javelin or else you will hit yourself in the back of the head." Get your whole body into the throw, and aim high to achieve the best distance.

Note

You're far from alone if you miss the target on the spear throw. Junyong says that he had to throw it three dozen times before figuring out the proper way to twist his wrist. And Margaret admits that the spear toss is her weakness: "I haven't made the throw yet in a race!"

Obstacle-Specific Training Exercises

Target Muscle Groups	Suggested Exercises
Primary	
Biceps	Chin-ups
Shoulders	Shoulder presses, lateral raises, reverse flies
Back	Dumbbell rows
Chest	Push-ups and any chest press variation preferably using dumbbells or barbells
Core	Torso rotations, bicycle maneuvers, abdominal Swiss ball crunches
Secondary	
Legs	Squats, lunges, calf raises

Tough Mudder's Electric Shock Station

Run through a field of live electric wires that deliver a jolt up to 10,000 volts.

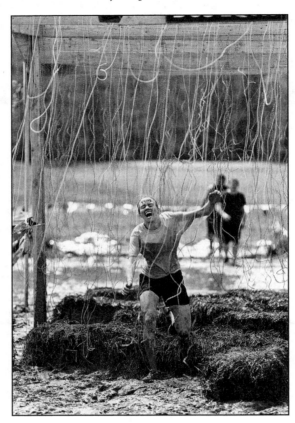

Plan to get zapped at Tough Mudder's Electric Shock Station.

(Dmitry Gudkov for Tough Mudder)

Expert Advice

If you're lucky, the wires hang far enough from the ground that you can crawl under them. If not, you don't have much choice but to "grin and bear it," according to Margaret.

With low-dangling wires, all of our experts recommend protecting your head and face by either wrapping your arms around your head and face, or using your arms to part the wires. Both techniques are intended to give your arms the brunt of the shock and protect your highly sensitive head and face. At that point, you can either "run like hell," as Joe likes to do, or take a slow, steady approach.

Amelia offers this weather-dependent tip: "If it's a windy day, watch where the wires are blowing and pick the area to run through that has the fewest wires (because the wind is blowing them away)."

Obstacle-Specific Training Exercises

Target Muscle Groups	Suggested Exercises
Primary	
Legs	Lunges, squats, calf raises
Heart/lungs	Sprinting or running
Secondary	
Core	Torso rotations, abdominal crunches, oblique crunches

Traverse Wall

Cling to the side of a wall and, using only small hand- and footholds, make your way from one end to the other.

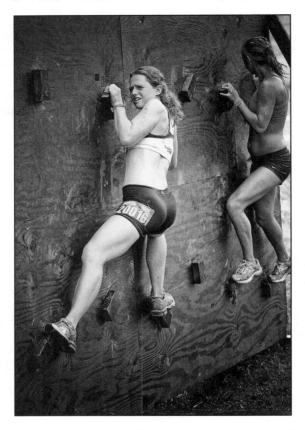

Try to keep your body as close to the traverse wall as possible to avoid falling off the tiny footholds.

(Photo courtesy of Nuvision Action Image)

Expert Advice

Hobie recommends keeping your body as close to the wall as you can, "as if you are a spider." This helps you stay balanced. Try not to let your hands get too close to your feet, or get your feet in front of your hands.

Grip strength is the key to success in this obstacle.

Obstacle-Specific Training Exercises

Target Muscle Groups	Suggested Exercises
Primary	
Hands and fingers	Finger flexion exercises such as tennis ball squeezes and grip master squeezes
Forearms	Hammer curls, reverse curls, hanging rope holds, forearm flexion and extension wrist curls
Legs	Leg curls, adductor machine, wide stance squats, stiff leg deadlifts
Biceps	Chin-ups
Secondary	
Serratus anterior	Straight arm pullovers
Trapezius	Shoulder shrugs

Wall Climbs

Scale walls and other barriers of various heights. Obstacles may be coated in mud, slime, or grease to make the challenge more difficult.

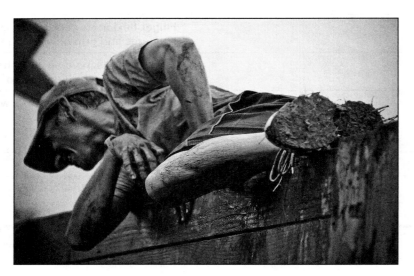

(Photo courtesy of Nuvision Action Image)

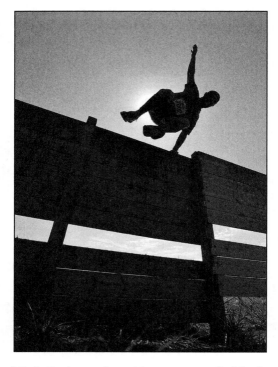

(Nick Graham photo/Courtesy Mudathlon)

Getting to the top of the wall obstacle is only half the battle at Spartan (top) and Mudathlon (bottom).
You also have to find a way back down.

Expert Advice

Make sure you have good footing and a good grip with your hands, and push up using your legs, while pulling using your arms. In some cases, you might need a helping hand (or boost) to get over the wall; don't be afraid to ask for assistance.

When you're near the top of the wall, don't try to get your feet over the wall first. Instead, bend over the wall at your waist, and let your feet follow. This technique takes the least amount of energy and lets you land softly on the other side.

Ever-resourceful, Hobie offers up this piece of practical advice: If walls are too tall to get over and nobody is around to help, sometimes you can use the posts holding the wall up as a step to boost yourself up.

Obstacle Ahead!

Don't climb a wall if you have an ankle, groin, or back injury.

Obstacle-Specific Training Exercises

Target Muscle Groups	Suggested Exercises
Primary	
Back	Pull-ups (close-grip to wide-grip variations, either assisted or full body and even with weight added)
Legs	Longer stride lunges (pushing back with the heels), standing and seated calf raises, squats, lunges
Secondary	
Forearm and biceps	Dumbbell hammer curls, reverse curl and neutral-grip pull-ups or pull-downs
Triceps	Triceps and chest dips, close-grip bench press, triceps push-downs
Shoulders	Shoulder presses, front shoulder raises

Water

Walk or swim through water. Often the water is chilly or freezing cold. Depths vary, but are usually not any more than chest-deep, allowing people who can't swim to walk or dog paddle across. Some water obstacles include barriers that you must crawl over or swim under to reach dry land.

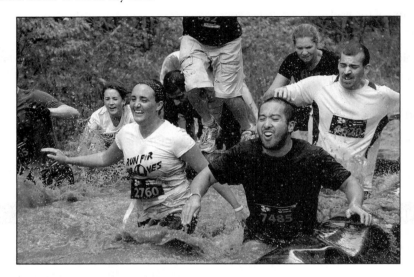

Plunging into frigid waters during the Run For Your Lives.

(Photo courtesy of Run For Your Lives)

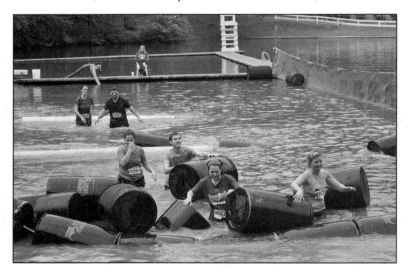

Racers avoid the many floating obstacles in Warrior Dash's Log Jam.

(Photo courtesy of Red Frog Events)

Expert Advice

According to Amelia, "Swims are typically not long and most of the time you can touch bottom. If you are not a stronger swimmer, walk as much as you can because swimming will tire you out. With extremely cold water, you will likely lose your breath when you first go in. Take a second to control your breathing—force yourself to take long, slow breaths."

Obstacle-Specific Training Exercises

Target Muscle Groups	Suggested Exercises
Back	Pull-ups (close-grip to wide-grip variations, either assisted or full body and even with weight added)
Core	Torso rotations, bicycle maneuvers, abdominal Swiss ball crunches
Legs	Longer stride lunges (pushing back with the heels), standing and seated calf raises, squats, lunges
Shoulders	Shoulder presses, front shoulder raises

Zombies

Try to avoid getting nabbed (or splattered) by zombies, paintball-gun-toting hillbillies, or other human obstacles. In Run For Your Lives, zombies chase participants as they navigate other obstacles in an attempt to snatch their "health flags" from them.

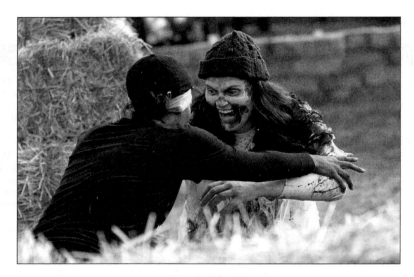

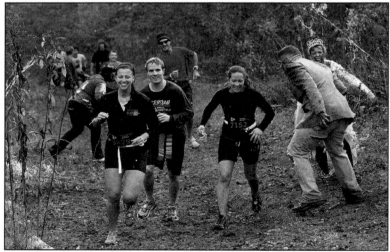

Zombies try to steal the runner's health flags in Run For Your Lives.

(Photos courtesy of Run For Your Lives)

Expert Advice

Run For Your Lives organizers passed along these hints for escaping the undead:

- Run with slower, less agile people, so zombies take their flags instead of yours.
- Run behind someone, using them as a shield against zombies.
- Run with large groups, so the zombies have lots of (other) targets.
- "Power spin" around the zombies—spinning flags are harder to grab.

Obstacle-Specific Training Exercises

Target Muscle Groups	Suggested Exercises
Legs	Lunges, squats, calf raises
Heart/lungs	Sprinting or running

Chapter 4

Race Attire for All Seasons

The performance gear industry makes mind-boggling amounts of money by convincing athletes—and athlete wannabes—that they need high-tech clothes and shoes to perform their best, and they make no exception when it comes to obstacle races. (Why else do you think several races are sponsored by gear companies?) And while it might be true that you can shave seconds off your time by wearing a specialized brand of shoes, shirt, and shorts instead of an old pair of sneakers, gym shorts, and a T-shirt, let me begin by saying that you don't need to go out and buy a whole new race-day wardrobe to successfully tackle an obstacle course race.

As a matter of fact, you probably shouldn't wear anything that's new, pricey, or fancy on race day because whatever you have on your bod is going to be trashed by the time you cross the finish line. Minimally, your clothes are going to be caked in mud, but they'll also likely get snagged on barbed wire or some other obstacle and be torn. Similarly, you might very well want to throw out (or recycle) your shoes—that is, if you still have them at the end of the race!

When selecting your race day attire you should focus on your comfort and safety. You also want to plan ahead for after the race, because you're going to want to change into clean, dry clothes for the postrace festivities and the drive home. Finally, you might want to pack your gear bag with some accessories that will enhance your experience, increase your safety, and enable you to document the adventure for your friends and family.

Clothes

Ideal warm-weather race-day attire is as follows:

- **A top** (optional) made of wicking material.
- **A sports bra** (females only); preferably the kind that you don't mind wearing without a shirt over it.
- **Shorts** that have a drawstring waistband or are tight enough to stay up on their own.
- **Socks** made of wool or synthetic fibers; wet cotton socks can chafe your feet and cause blisters.
- **Underwear** made of nylon or other synthetic material that wicks moisture away from your skin. Not only is wet cotton uncomfortable, but it can cause chafing.

For colder weather (50°F or below), you may want to trade in the shorts for running capris or tights and layer on an additional top. Don't go overboard with the layers, though, because once you get out on the course your body temperature will go a long way to keeping you warm, and you don't have to haul a bunch of sopping wet layers with you.

Keep in mind that if you do plan to keep your clothes, you should probably wear dark colors to hide the stains. White or other light-colored clothes may look dingy no matter how many times you wash them.

Here are some dos and don'ts of dressing for an obstacle course race:

- *Do* **wear a lightweight material, such as spandex, lycra, CoolMax, or Dri-Fit, that wicks away moisture.** The corollary to this rule is to avoid wearing cotton, as it retains moisture. Not only are you going to sweat, but most courses have water features that will soak you from head to toe.
- *Don't* **wear excessively baggy clothes.** Baggy clothes are far more likely to get caught on barbed wire, branches, and other obstacles, and they will also sag and weigh you down when you get wet. Tight-fitting shorts also minimize the possibility of an embarrassing pants mishap on the course.
- *Do* **pack a spare set of clothes to change into after the race.** Don't forget dry underwear and socks.
- *Don't* **wear clothes with pockets.** They will fill with mud, muck, and water and weigh you down on the course.

- ***Don't* wear anything that you don't want to get ruined.** Whatever you have on is going to get dirty and potentially ripped or torn. Save the pricey duds for after the race.

Everything from your gear bag down to your shoes are going to be a wet, stinky mess. That includes a camera, so if you want to snap photos during the challenge, take an inexpensive model that's small enough to fit inside a plastic sandwich bag that can tuck into your shirt or pocket (but see the bullet on pockets earlier in this section).

Obstacle Ahead!

Avoid wearing cotton clothes such as hooded sweatshirts, sweatpants, and even T-shirts made out of cotton. On chilly days wet cotton can keep you chilled because the fabric doesn't wick moisture away from your skin. Loose, wet cotton is also more likely than many other fabrics to chafe, and few things during a race are as uncomfortable as red, raw thighs, arms, and bra line (for gals) or nipples (for guys) from chafing.

Athletic swimwear, either as a layer or complete outfit, presents a practical option if the course includes water obstacles or mud pits. But if you wear relatively tight-fitting clothing, you can jump in without having to change.

Planning to wear a costume? Follow the same principles outlined in this section: select close-fitting material that wicks away moisture. Also, try to keep accessories to a minimum so you don't have to haul them with you over, under, and through the obstacles. A cape, hat, or other accessory that you don't have to hold on to should be fine (although they might get blown off or snagged on an obstacle), but anything that you have to carry around is going to be a headache when you need both of your hands for tackling the obstacles.

Shoes

Yes, you do need to wear shoes. No bare feet, and no army boots. The terrain at many courses can include sharp rocks and sticks, which can injure bare feet. Boots aren't recommended because of the damage they can do to the course and other participants. And when boots get wet, they soak up a lot of water, increasing the weight you'll be carrying around for the rest of the race.

Preferably, you want to wear shoes that you won't mind throwing away (most races actually offer to recycle them) at the finish line after they're soaked in mud, or that you can easily clean. If you have an old pair of trail running shoes, you have an ideal pair of race shoes. Just as with clothes, loose shoes can get lost in the mud. Keep the laces tied tightly. Some participants recommend wrapping duct tape around the top of the shoe and ankle to keep it on your feet, but this can reduce traction; instead, double-tie your laces and tuck the ends under the tongue.

Here are some characteristics of an ideal pair of obstacle race shoes:

- **Lightweight,** so as not to absorb a lot of water on the course
- **Tight-fitting,** so it will be less likely to be sucked off in the mud
- **Good traction** for slippery terrain
- **Relatively thick soles** to handle rocks and roots

Of course, everyone's feet are different, so you should pick a pair of shoes that you know you'll be comfortable in even when they get wet. Some runners need heavier shoes due to bad arches or other foot problems.

Obstacle Ahead!

Never wear a pair of shoes for the first time during the race—that's a recipe for race-day disaster. Make sure you try out the shoes on the types of terrain you'll be racing on. That means over rough, rocky trails, through thick sand and mud, and in the water. Only wear specialized shoes like Vibram FiveFingers if you've been training in them for at least a few weeks. They take some getting used to, and you'll have enough to worry about on the course without having to struggle with blisters or sore feet.

You'll need a pair of postrace shoes, too. Flip-flops or sandals that can get dirty make it easy to stroll around the postrace party while protecting your feet.

Specialized Gear

You'll see participants carrying just about everything under the sun to give themselves an extra edge at obstacle races. Although Spartan has let people carry a length of rope, Joe Desena of Spartan Race said he's seen one person try to bring a ladder onto the course. "Obviously not allowed."

But Amit Nar, founder of Rebel Race, begged to differ. "I haven't had anyone bring a ladder," he said, laughing. "But they could if they wanted to! But then they've got to lug the ladder all the way through. Some people bring a medicine ball and carry it all the way through, just for the extra challenge."

Although I certainly don't recommend strapping a ladder on your back—or carrying a medicine ball, for that matter—some specialized equipment might come in handy, particularly if the weather is cold.

Tip

Add cheap foam shin guards or elbow pads to your gear list—they come in very handy on crawls!

Wetsuits

Top racer Junyong Pak reports that he gets a lot of questions from people wondering if they should wear a wetsuit. "Every single [Tough Mudder] has a cold element involved, such as dumpsters filled with chunks of ice floating in water. People tend to think they need to protect themselves from the cold, but you don't want to overprotect yourself. You can overcome the cold by working hard enough and moving enough—without needing a wetsuit. You can suffer heat stroke on even a mountainous course if you wear a wetsuit; it almost happened to me."

Gloves

Although wetsuits might be overkill, gloves can come in handy, particularly during cold weather and if you're serious about shaving seconds off your time. They provide extra grip on obstacles, such as the monkey bars, that might be greased and will probably be slippery with mud from other racers. However, once the gloves get wet, they add extra weight and can keep you chilled. And if your hands and forearms are chilled, you lose dexterity, which hurts your grip.

Along the same lines, Junyong Pak suggests protecting your forearms somehow. "Only recently had an 'aha' moment. If I had neoprene sleeves—I'd cut off sleeves from wetsuit but lost them—it would've been a huge plus to use to cover forearms," he said.

Tip

For cold-weather races or if your hands tend to get chilled quickly, consider investing in a pair of neoprene paddling gloves. Not only do these gloves usually have a rubberized outer layer, which provides extra grip (perfect for rope climbs and monkey bars), but they are usually waterproof and cinch at the wrist, which helps keeps the water away from your skin.

Race-Day Packing List

This may seem like a lot of stuff to stash into your gear bag, but with the exception of the camera and watch, it really is the bare minimum you should pack:

- ❏ **Photo ID:** For checking in.

- ❏ **Plastic bottles of water:** Although the races provide water stations during the race, you'll want water or sports drinks to hydrate before and after the race. Keep in mind, however, that some races won't let you bring any liquids onto the site, instead requiring you to purchase water from their vendors.

- ❏ **Bug spray:** Mosquitoes, gnats, black flies, and other biting insects can serve as extra obstacles on the course.

- ❏ **Sunscreen:** You can get burned even on cool, overcast days.

- ❏ **Registration forms and waiver:** You should download and print these forms in advance (just don't forget to bring them with you!).

- ❏ **Waterproof watch:** Even if you don't care about your race time, you'll want to have a watch so you can make it to the start on time for your heat.

- ❏ **Small first aid kit:** You'll want to keep this in your car in case you need antibacterial cream and bandages for minor cuts.

- ❏ **Plastic bags:** To carry your dirty clothes home.

- ❏ **Dark towels:** For cleaning up and to sit on during the drive home.

- ❏ **Wet wipes:** To clean your face and hands.

- ❏ **Blankets, lawn chairs, shade umbrella:** For after the race.

- ❏ **Cash:** For food, beverages, and souvenirs at the postrace party.

- ❏ **Extra clothes and shoes:** To change into for the postrace festivities. This includes a clean top, bottom, bra (for women), underwear, and socks. Even if it's supposed to be a warm day, bring plenty of warm layers, as you might be chilled after the race.

- ❏ **Old camera:** For snapping pix of you and your friends. Another great option is to wear a POV camera (head cam) like a GoPro so you capture yourself conquering the obstacles on film.

- ❏ **A great attitude!** You should never travel to any race (or anywhere, for that matter) without it.

Tip

If you wear prescription glasses, attach them to your head using a sports band or eyewear retainer.

Although I don't recommend wearing goggles during the race, if you wear contact lenses, bring along some eye drops or saline to rinse them of dirt particles after the race.

Gear Check

What should you do with all your extra gear—the change of clothes, cash, and towel—while you're racing? You can leave it stashed with a buddy who came to watch or locked in your car, but most races have a gear check station where you can store your stuff while you're on the course.

What Not to Bring

Don't make the first-timer mistake of bringing along possessions that are going to either get you in trouble with race staff or that will be a hassle to have with you on race day:

- **iPod:** You'd be surprised how many first-time racers show up thinking they can run with their iPod. Leave it in the car or at home. It will get ruined on the course.
- **Sunglasses:** Just as with the iPod, you're likely to lose them; however, you might want to have a pair in your gear bag to wear after the race.
- **Jewelry:** Ditto. This applies even—maybe even especially—to wedding rings.
- **Pets:** They aren't allowed on the course and will be miserable in the car on a hot day, so don't bother.

Chapter 5

Lower-Body
Exercises

Gluteus maximus. No, it's not the name of an ancient Roman conqueror, but it is going to help you conquer your next obstacle race. The largest of a trio of muscles (for the record, the other two are the gluteus medius and the gluteus minimus) that comprise your buttocks, the gluteus maximus is one of the most powerful muscles in the human body. And if I had to pick just one muscle to focus on when training for an obstacle race, I'd choose the glutes. That's because they're the major source of propulsive force for your body. *Translation:* you need them to move forward. The stronger your glutes, the more quickly and powerfully you can run, jump, and leap.

But just because your glutes are king doesn't mean you should ignore the rest of the muscles in your lower body. These include your quads and hamstrings in your upper legs and your calves in your lower legs, as well as a host of smaller muscles. All of your lower-body muscles work together to serve as your foundation and the source of almost all of your forward movements.

Crawls, climbs, leaps, and hurdles all require a strong lower body. Even obstacles that primarily tax the upper body or core—such as the spear throw, rope climb, and carry and hauls—require lower-body strength for peak performance.

And then, of course, there's the running component of all obstacle races. Strong leg muscles not only propel you forward more quickly, they also help protect joints that can take a beating on the course.

Oh, and by the way, all the new-fangled training regimens and fad exercises in the world can't beat good old-fashioned squats and lunges for strengthening the lower body, so I include a lot of variations on those two themes in this chapter.

Finally, here are some tips to keep in mind when training:

- Use a full range of motion on all exercises.
- Lift weights and perform calisthenics at a moderate pace.
- Don't jerk or bounce weights—let the muscles do the work.
- Be mindful of the muscles you're working before, during, and after you train. Doing so will lead to better muscle stimulation and, ultimately, a much better workout.

Dumbbell Squat

1. **Grasp two dumbbells and allow your arms to hang down by your sides, palms facing your hips.**

    Alternatively, you can hold the weights shoulder height with your elbows bent and your palms facing your chest.

2. **Assume a shoulder-width stance, and slowly lower your body until your thighs are approximately parallel to the ground.**

    Your lower back should be slightly arched and your heels should stay in contact with the floor at all times.

3. **When you reach a "seated" position, reverse direction by pressing through the heels while straightening your legs until you return to the start position.**

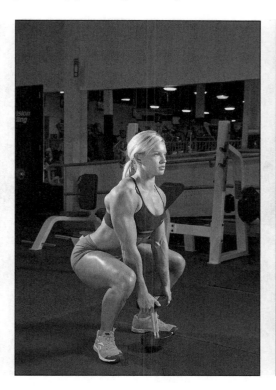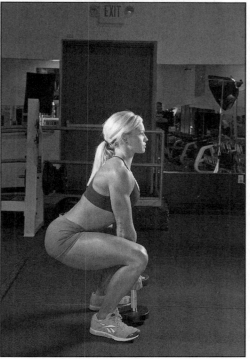

Tip

For all squats, your breathing should follow a regular pattern: inhale as you lower your body and exhale as you raise yourself back up to a standing position.

Dumbbell Sumo Squat

1. **Grasp two dumbbells and allow your arms to hang down by your sides, palms facing your hips.**

   Alternatively, hold the weights shoulder height with your elbows bent and your palms facing your chest.

2. **Assume a wider than shoulder-width stance, and slowly lower your body until your thighs are approximately parallel to the ground.**

   Your lower back should be slightly arched and your heels should stay in contact with the floor at all times.

3. **When you reach a "seated" position, reverse direction by pressing through the heels while straightening your legs until you return to the start position.**

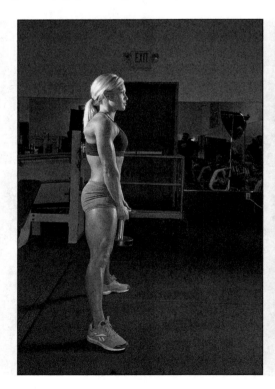
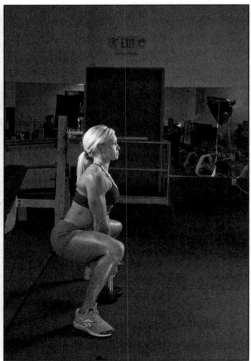

Dumbbell Pilates Squat

1. **Grasp two dumbbells and allow your arms to hang down by your sides with your palms facing your hips.**

   Alternatively, hold the weights shoulder height with your elbows bent and your palms facing your chest.

2. **Assume a wider than shoulder-width stance with your toes pointed out 45 degrees and then slowly lower your body while pushing your knees toward your toes.**

   Your upper body should be tall and your heels should stay in contact with the floor.

3. **When you reach a comfortable low position, reverse direction by pressing through the heels while straightening your legs until you return to the start position.**

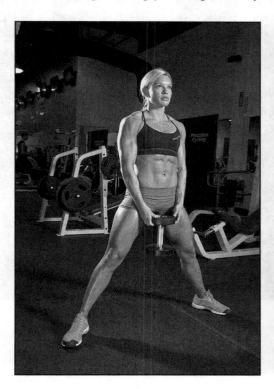 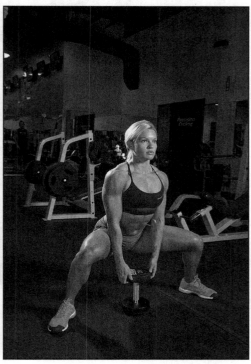

Note

Athletes tend to get tight glutes, quads, and hamstrings, which can lead to strains and even tears. The best way to avoid these injuries is to maintain your flexibility by stretching the muscles regularly. Head over to Chapter 10 for stretching exercises you should do after every workout.

Dumbbell Calf Raises

1.   Stand on a step (or staircase) and allow your heels to drop below your toes.

2.   Hold onto a stationary object with one hand and hold a dumbbell in the other hand.

3.   Slowly rise as high as you can onto your toes until your calves are fully flexed.

4.   Contract your calves and then slowly reverse direction until you return to the starting position.

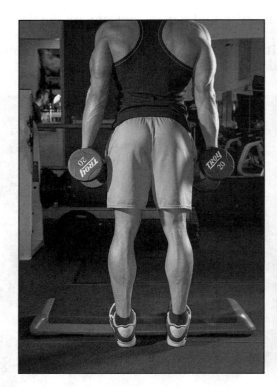 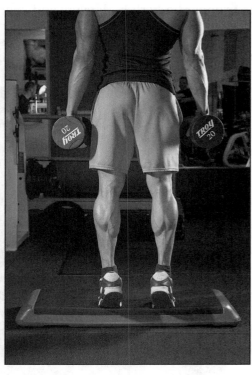

Side Lying Leg Raises

1. Lie on your left side, bend your left leg at a 90-degree angle, and bring your left foot to rest underneath your right knee.

2. Keeping your right leg straight, slowly raise it as high as possible while pointing the toe down and heel up.

3. Contract your glutes, and then slowly return along the same path back to the start position.

4. After finishing the desired number of repetitions, repeat the process on your left.

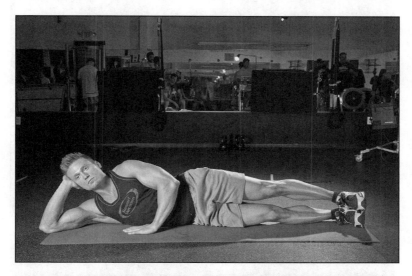

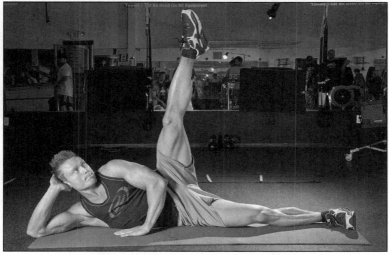

Tip

You can make this exercise more challenging by using ankle weights.

Butt Hip Raises

1. Lie on your back with your knees bent at 90 degrees and your hands on the floor at your side.

2. Press through your heels and raise your hips toward the ceiling while contracting your glute muscles.

3. Lower your hips and release the glute contraction.

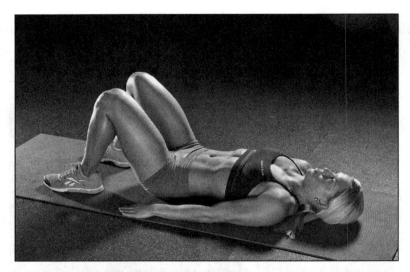

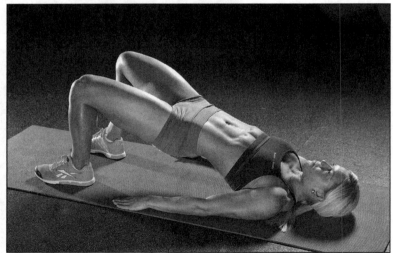

Dumbbell Back Lunges

1.   Grasp two dumbbells and allow them to hang down by your sides.

2.   Take a long stride backward with your right leg and keep your left heel down.

3.   Keeping your shoulders back and chin up, slowly lower your body by flexing your knees and hip, continuing your descent until your right knee almost touches the floor.

    Make sure that your left knee does not go past your toes.

4.   Reverse direction by forcibly extending your left hip and knee until you return to the start position.

5.   After performing the desired number of reps, repeat the process on your right.

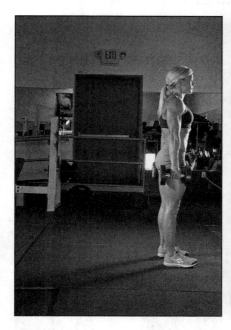 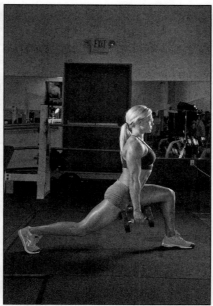 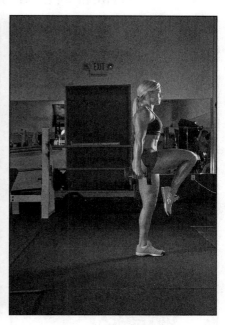

Note

You get a bonus for training your lower-body muscles: a natural boost in your body's natural fat-burning growth hormones. Because your lower-body muscles are so large, when you give them a good workout, you generate larger quantities of growth hormones than you do when you work out your upper body. The more muscle mass you have, the more growth hormone you send coursing through your body when you work out!

Dumbbell Forward Lunges

1. Grasp two dumbbells and allow them to hang down by your sides.

2. Take a long stride forward with your right leg and raise your left heel so that your left foot is on its toes.

3. Keeping your shoulders back and chin up, slowly lower your body by flexing your knees and hip, continuing your descent until your left knee almost touches the floor.

    Make sure that your right knee does not go past your toes.

4. Reverse direction by forcibly extending the right hip and knee until you return to the start position.

5. After performing the desired number of reps, repeat the process on your left.

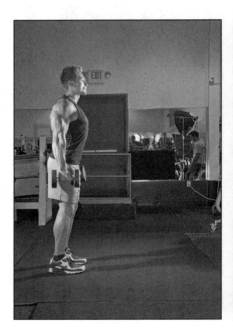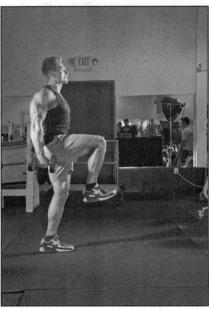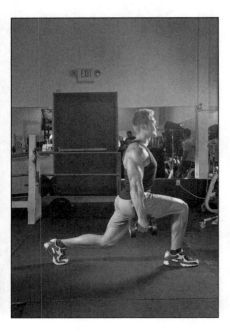

Dumbbell Back Diagonal Lunges

1. Grasp two dumbbells and allow them to hang down by your sides.

2. Take a long diagonal stride back with your right leg toward your left side and turn your left foot inward.

3. Keeping your shoulders back and chin up, slowly lower your body by flexing your knees and hip, continuing your descent until your left knee is almost in contact with the floor.

    Make sure that your left knee does not go past your toes.

4. Reverse direction by forcibly extending the left hip and knee until you return to the start position.

5. After performing the desired number of reps, repeat the process on your right.

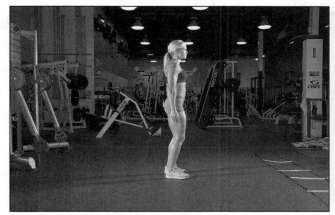 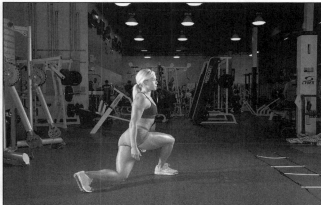

Tip

Ankle strains and sprains are some of the most common injuries people suffer while preparing for and participating in obstacle races. Physical therapist Michael Camp says that the key to strengthening your ankle is proprioception: work on unstable surfaces by exercising on foam mats, wobble boards, and balance boards. You don't even need equipment to strengthen your ankle; all you need is a partner to toss you a medicine ball while you stand on one leg and catch it.

Bonus Workout: Hobie Call's Weight Vest Training

Unlike regular running, where you're just running down a road, in obstacle races you'll be running off-road through mud and water, up and down steep hills, and having to complete a series of obstacles along the way. Your pace will be slower, and lower-body strength will play a much greater role in success. This is why I wear a weight vest when I train. It provides "functional" skeletal and muscular resistance. I say functional, because you can also do heavy squats to build extra skeletal and muscular strength, but heavy squats don't convert to faster running. A weight vest is a functional training device, because it doesn't alter your biomechanics.

When it comes to how much weight to put in the vest, you want to find that happy medium where you can feel the resistance, but it doesn't slow you down too much. For the races I'm training for now, I wear 10 pounds. When I was training for the Spartan Death Race, I did this workout with 30 pounds. I wore more for the Death Race, because strength was a much bigger factor than speed.

Lunges are also great, because they allow you to work your muscles harder than you would otherwise be able to do while also working them through a full range of motion, helping to keep you flexible. I alternate doing butt kickers with high knees, which helps activate my hamstrings and hip flexors, while also increasing their range of motion.

Aerobically, I run at the same intensity that I would a tempo run (see Chapter 11), but with the lunges thrown in, my legs get a far better workout than they otherwise could. This helps with the extra strength required when carrying logs/tires/buckets/sandbags, etc.

For more tips from Hobie, check out his obstacle race training videos at conqueranycourse.com.

Chapter 6

Upper-Body Exercises

The upper body includes the muscles of the arms, chest, shoulders, upper back, neck, and hands. That's a lot of body parts and associated muscles, and you'll need every one of them on the obstacle course.

If you have a strong upper body, you can ease some of the stress on your lower body when tackling many of the obstacles. Instead of relying exclusively on your legs and glutes to thrust yourself upward and over hurdles and walls, you can draw on your upper-body strength to pull yourself up and over. Similarly, you'll find yourself using your arms and shoulders almost as much as you do your legs on low crawls. And forearm strength is key for getting through monkey bars and wall traverse.

If you can use your upper-body strength to supplement your lower body and core on the obstacles, you'll be able to save up more energy in your legs for the running portion of the course.

Dumbbell Chest Press

1. Lay face up on a flat bench with your feet planted firmly on the floor.

2. Grasp two dumbbells and, with your palms facing away from your body, bring the weights to shoulder level so that they rest just above your armpits.

3. Simultaneously press both dumbbells directly over your chest, moving them in toward each other on the ascent. At the finish of the movement, the sides of the dumbbells should gently touch together.

    You should feel a contraction in your chest muscles at the top of the movement.

4. Slowly reverse direction, returning to the starting position.

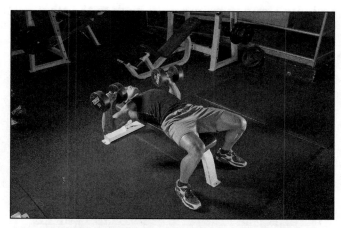

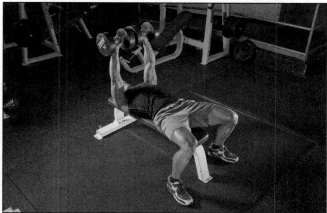

Note

When lifting weights, the negative portion of the repetition (when you're lowering the weight) should take longer then the concentric (when you're raising the weight). It is easier to lower a weight than lift it, so by lowering it in a controlled manner and at a slower speed, you recruit more muscle fibers and get more work done.

Dumbbell Chest Flies

1. **Lay back on a flat bench, planting your feet firmly on the floor.**

2. **Grasp two dumbbells and bring them out to your sides, maintaining a slight bend to your elbows throughout the move.**

   Your palms should be facing in and toward the ceiling, and your upper arms should be roughly parallel with the level of the bench.

3. **Slowly raise the weights upward in a semicircular motion, as if you're hugging a large tree, and gently touch the weights together at the top of the move.**

   You should feel a contraction in your chest muscles at the top of the move.

4. **Slowly return the weights along the same path back to the start position.**

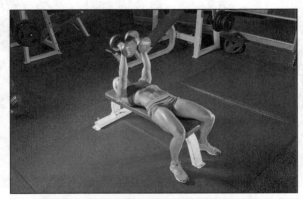

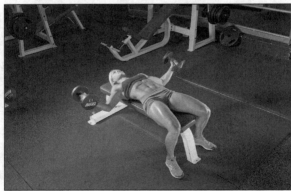

Note

When doing strength-training exercises, your breathing should follow a certain pattern. You want to exhale on exertion, or when the muscle is contracting, and then inhale as you relax, or when the muscle is elongating. For example, when doing a biceps curl, exhale as you curl (or bend) your elbow, and then inhale when you lower (or extend) your elbow.

Dumbbell Incline Chest Press

1. Lay face up on an incline bench angled at approximately 30 to 40 degrees, and plant your feet firmly on the floor.

2. Grasp two dumbbells and, with your palms facing away from your body, bring the weights to shoulder level so that they rest just above your armpits.

3. Simultaneously press both dumbbells directly over your chest, moving them in toward each other on the ascent.

   At the finish of the movement, the sides of the dumbbells should gently touch together. You should feel a contraction in your chest muscles at the top of the movement.

4. Slowly reverse direction, returning to the starting position.

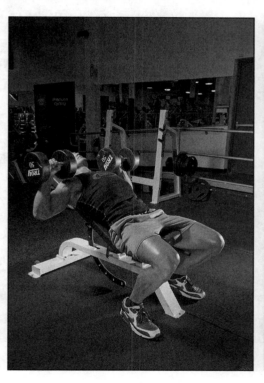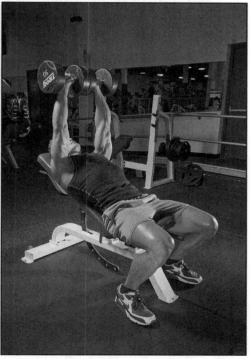

Obstacle Ahead!

When you are engaged in a set of exercises, try to avoid taking mini breaks at the start position. The optimal way to recruit muscle fibers is to keep that muscle under tension for the duration of the set. If you are going super heavy and need to catch your breath, a small rest may work for you, but if you need to rest, you should probably use a slightly lighter weight and try to push through without stopping.

Dumbbell Biceps Curl

1. **Stand with soft knees and relaxed shoulders.**

2. **Grasp two dumbbells and allow the weights to hang at your sides with your hands facing away from your body.**

    Press your elbows into your sides and keep them stable throughout the move.

3. **Simultaneously, slowly curl both dumbbells up toward your shoulders and contract your biceps at the top of the move.**

4. **Slowly reverse direction and return to the start position.**

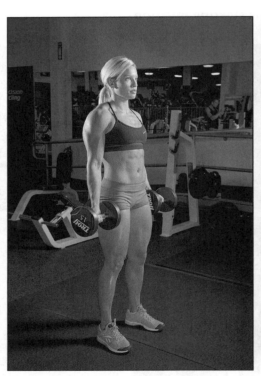 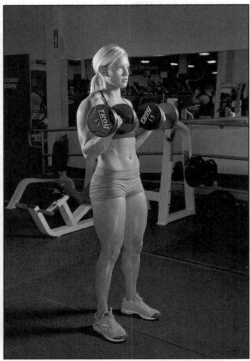

Tip

When it comes to choosing the correct weight, here's the deal: It's about going on a discovery of your lifting and limit patterns. Choose a weight that you know you can handle, master that exercise's form and your anatomical position, and perform eight repetitions. Once you're completely comfortable with the lift and the weight you've chosen, increase the weight in 5-pound increments.

Dumbbell Incline Biceps Curl

1. Lay back on a 45-degree incline bench.

2. Grasp two dumbbells and allow the weights to hang by your hips with your palms facing forward.

3. Keeping your upper arm stable, slowly curl the dumbbells upward toward your shoulders.

    Make sure your elbows stay back throughout the movement.

4. Contract your biceps and then slowly return the weights to the starting position.

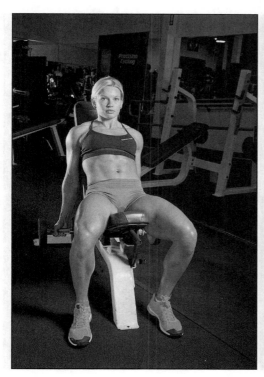 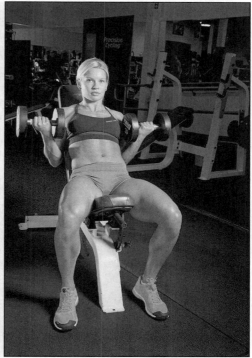

Note

In my 22 years of training, I've noticed that women tend to *underestimate* the weight of the dumbbell they can handle while men tend to choose weights that are *too heavy* for their abilities. So ladies, I encourage you to up your weights and really see what you're made of. And gents, you might want to back off a few pounds and increase the number of reps instead.

Dumbbell Triceps Overhead Extension

1.   Stand upright with your knees slightly bent.

2.   Grasp two dumbbells and raise your arms overhead and shoulder-width apart.

3.   With your palm facing each other, lower the weights down toward your shoulder.

     Keep elbows pointing forward and in front so you can see them out of the corners of your eyes.

4.   Reverse direction and return the weights back to the starting position.

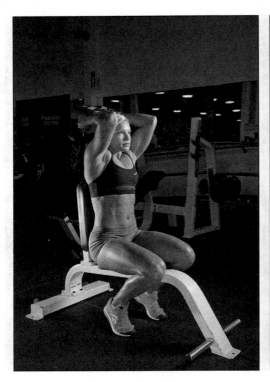 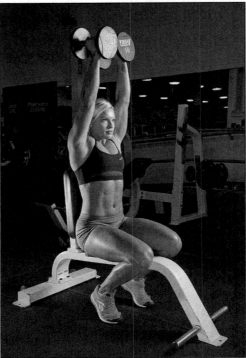

Obstacle Ahead!

Don't get caught up in the bodybuilder mentality of thinking you need huge biceps and a ripped chest to succeed on the obstacle course. Functional strength—the ability to actually complete various tasks on the course—is far more important than being able to bench press a certain weight. It's also better to do more reps at a lower weight than to do fewer at a higher weight.

Dumbbell Triceps Kick Back

1. Stand with your body bent forward at the waist so that your torso is virtually parallel with the ground.

2. Grasp two dumbbells and raise your elbows back as high as possible.

3. With your palm facing your body, raise the weights by extending your elbows until it is parallel with the floor.

4. Reverse direction and return the weights back to the starting position.

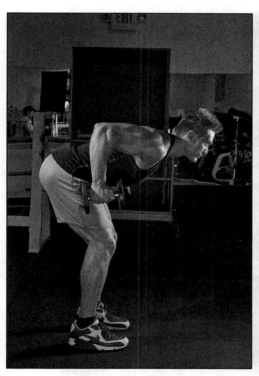 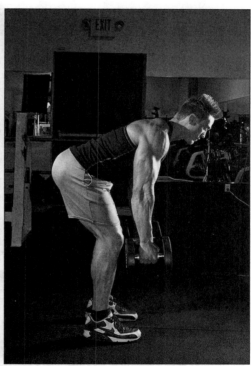

Dumbbell Triceps Skull Crusher

1. Lay back on a flat bench with your feet planted firmly on the floor.

2. Grasp two dumbbells with your palms facing each other and straighten your arms so that the weights are directly over your chest.

3. Keeping your elbows in and pointed toward the ceiling, slowly lower the weights toward your ears and pause at this point.

4. Extend your elbows so that the weights return to your starting position.

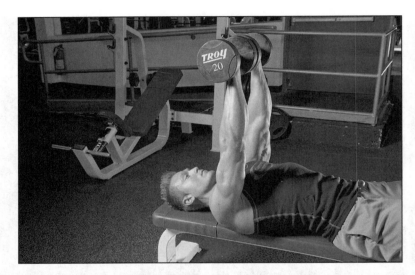

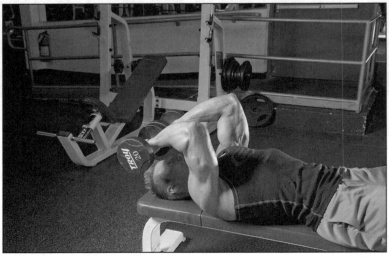

Dumbbell Back Flies

1. **Stand with your body bent forward at the waist so that your torso is virtually parallel with the ground.**

    Your torso should remain parallel with the ground throughout the entire exercise.

2. **Grasp two dumbbells with your palms facing each other, and let the weights hang down to the ground.**

3. **With slightly bent elbows, raise the weights laterally away from the center of your body until your arms are shoulder height.**

    You should feel a contraction in the muscles between your shoulder blades.

4. **Reverse direction, lowering the dumbbells along the same path back to your starting position.**

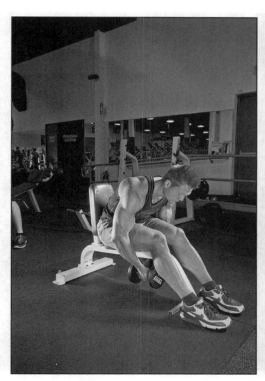 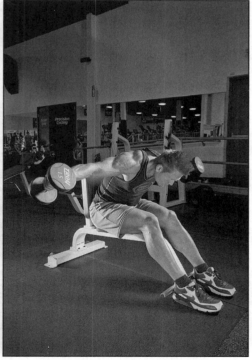

Dumbbell Back Rows

1. **Stand with your body bent forward at the waist so that your torso is virtually parallel with the ground.**

   Your torso should remain parallel with the ground throughout the entire movement.

2. **Grasp two dumbbells with your palms facing each other, and let the weights hang down to the ground.**

3. **Keeping your elbows close to your body, pull the dumbbells upward and back until they touch your hip or lower stomach area.**

   You should feel a contraction in the muscles of your upper back.

4. **Reverse direction, lowering the dumbbells along the same path back to the starting position.**

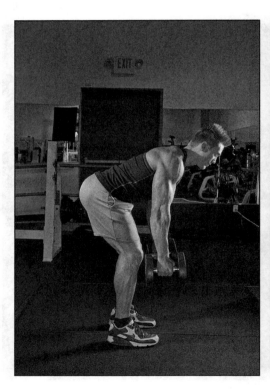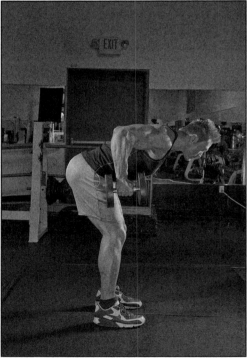

Dumbbell Shoulder Press

1. Grasp two dumbbells and stand with your knees slightly bent.

2. Bring the weights to shoulder level with your palms facing away from your body.

3. Slowly press the dumbbells directly upward and in, allowing them to touch together directly over your head.

4. Contract your deltoids and then slowly return the dumbbells along the same arc back to the start position.

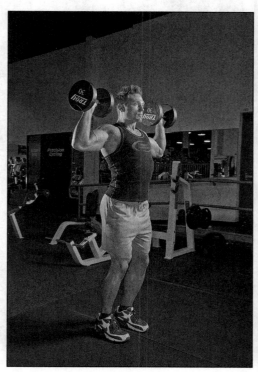 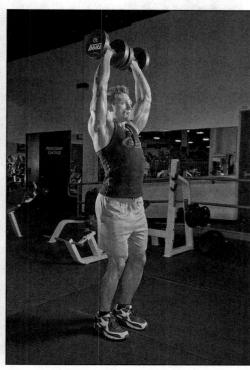

Dumbbell Deltoid Lateral Raise

1. **Grasp two dumbbells, allowing them to hang by your hips.**

2. **With a slight bend to your elbows, raise the weights up and out to the sides until they reach shoulder level.**

    At the top of the movement, the rear of the dumbbells should be slightly higher than the front.

3. **Slowly return the weights back to the starting position.**

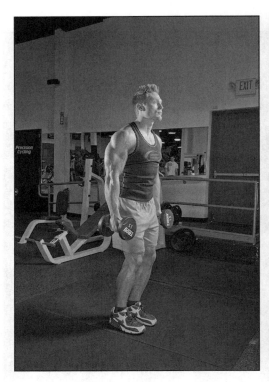 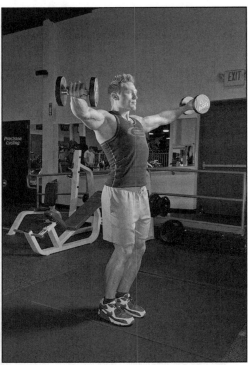

Dumbbell Deltoid Frontal Raise

1. **Grasp two dumbbells, allowing them to hang by your hips.**

    Your palms should face inward, toward your body.

2. **With a slight bend to your elbows, slowly raise the weights directly in front of your body until they reach shoulder level.**

3. **Contract your deltoids at the top of the movement, and then slowly return the weights to the starting position.**

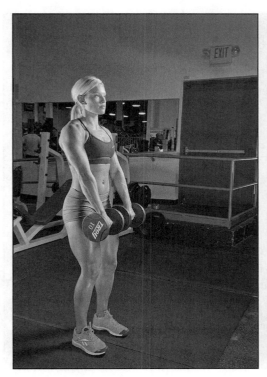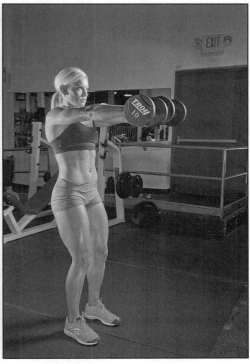

Triceps Dips

1. Place your heels on the floor and your hands on the edge of a flat bench, keeping your arms straight.

2. Slowly bend your elbows as far as comfortably possible, allowing your butt to descend below the level of the bench.

   Make sure your elbows stay close to your body throughout the move.

3. Reverse direction and straighten your arms, returning to the start position.

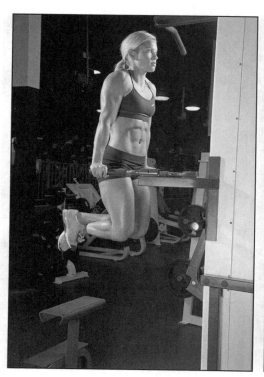 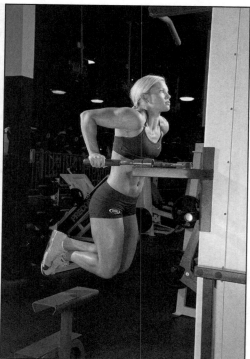

Tip

Champion obstacle course racer Junyong Pak says that after cardio fitness he places the most emphasis on forearm strength. According to Pak, when people fail at an obstacle, it's often because of weak or tired forearms. To develop forearm strength, Pak recommends doings lots of pull-ups and push-ups, and even just hanging from a bar to build up your grip and forearm. When you're able to hang on for at least a minute, go to the advanced level by coating the bar with mud to simulate the realities of the obstacle course.

Chest Dips

1. **Grasp the handles of a dip station or dip machine, extend your arms, and lock them at the elbows.**

2. **Align your body so that your head, upper and lower body, and feet are in a single plane.**

3. **Bend your legs at the knees and hook your feet over one another.**

   This position helps keep your back arched and your chest muscles engaged.

4. **Slowly lower yourself by bending your elbows, leaning your head and upper body forward as you make your descent.**

   The farther you lean forward, the more your chest muscles will work. Keep your elbows and arms away from your body to better isolate the chest muscles and avoid recruiting the triceps.

5. **Lower yourself until the backs of your upper arms are parallel or slightly beyond parallel with the floor.**

   Never go so low that you feel any chest or shoulder pain or you could seriously injure yourself.

6. **When you reach the bottom position, do not rest. Instead, slowly begin to press your body upward without using any momentum.**

   Make sure that you maintain your postural alignment.

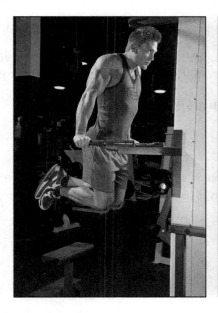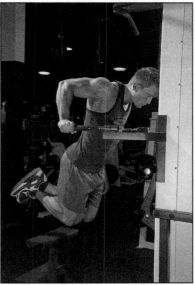

Tip

As you near the top of the motion, your goal is not to lock out the elbows or triceps but instead to contract and squeeze the chest muscles as hard as you possibly can for a two-second count.

Bonus Upper-Body Workout: Hobie Call's Rock Training

This is a full-body workout with the primary focus on your upper body. If you don't want to use a rock, you can use a medicine ball, fitness sand bag, or any other heavy object.

You want a rock that you can lift above your head without struggling and can throw at least 10 feet. Ultimately, you want to lift between 20 and 40 pounds. If you have to start with less than 20 pounds that's fine, but focus on building your strength until you can handle at least 20 pounds. If 40 pounds isn't hard enough, don't go heavier; instead, incorporate a weight vest into the workout. Too much weight will just make your arms so large that your running will suffer, and that's not very efficient training for obstacle racing. I personally like to do this workout with a 30-pound rock.

Treat the first set as your warm-up, so take it easy on this round.

1.   **Set your stopwatch for two minutes (have it set so it will start over every two minutes). Start your timer.**

2.   **Pick up the rock, curl it up to your chest, and throw it straight out in front of you.**

       Continue throwing the rock until the timer goes off.

3.   **When the timer goes off, do 10 push-ups. For the remainder of the two minutes, pick up the rock and throw it backward over your head.**

       If push-ups are too easy, do dive bombers.

4.   **When the timer goes off, do 10 burpees and then pick the rock up, lift it above your head, and throw it down just a few feet in front of you (focusing on the downward force).**

       If you're near a spot where you can do pull-ups, mix them in with the push-ups and burpees.

5.   **When the timer goes off, do 10 push-ups again. Then holding the rock at your waist, curl the rock and go straight into a shoulder press. Repeat that until the timer goes off.**

6.   **Continue the eight-minute cycle (steps 1 through 5) three to five times.**

Tip

You want this workout to be cardiovascularly intense, so if you need to, run between throws or if you want it to be more upper body intense, do things like army crawl to the rock after you throw it.

Chapter 7

Functional and Compound Exercises

Spend any time with obstacle racers and you'll probably hear the phrase *functional training* tossed around quite a bit. That's because functional training is a way to train for the rigors of the obstacle course racing by mimicking the actual movements you need to perform on the course. Functional training involves harnessing the body's full range of motion in your workouts. So instead of using fixed-plane machines to do your shoulder presses, back flies, leg extensions, and so on, functional exercises work those same muscle groups but also require you to maintain the balance and appropriate plane of movement you need to focus on those muscles. In other words, functional exercises work the peripheral muscles that help stabilize a joint; single-plane exercises don't.

Studies show that functional training techniques not only improve strength over fixed workouts, but also significantly increase balance and reduce the likelihood of joint pain. For example, although many single-plane exercises can increase the strength of the rotator cuff, they rarely focus on the scapula stabilizers around the rotator cuff. To prevent injury to the rotator cuff, you need strong scapula stabilizers. By focusing on both the rotator cuff and scapula stabilizers, functional exercises can result in fewer injuries and an overall stronger body.

Equipment used in functional training include dumbbells, kettlebells, sandbags, resistance tubes, exercise balls, and suspension systems such as Total Body Resistance Exercise or TRX.

The second half of this chapter focuses on compound exercises, which are exercises that work more than one muscle group or joint.

TRX Suspended Leg Circles

1. Lie on your stomach and insert your toes in the TRX toe loops.

2. Raise your upper body into a push-up (keep your hands shoulder-width apart) or elbow plank position.

3. Pull both knees in, and then circle them away from the center of your body.

    Your legs will meet in the center, in an extended plank position.

4. Repeat steps 1 through 3.

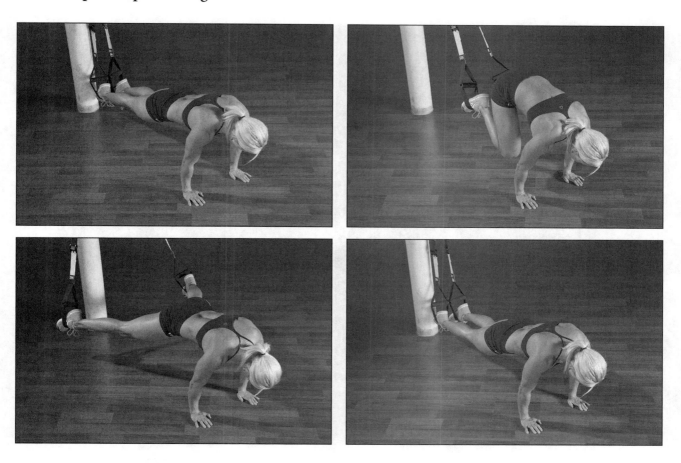

Note

Suspension training is a type of resistance training that uses ropes or straps to harness the body's own weight to perform multiplane movements. TRX is the most popular brand of suspension training system.

TRX Suspended V Pike

1. Lie on your stomach and insert your toes in the TRX toe loops.

2. Raise your upper body into a push-up (keep your hands shoulder-width apart) or elbow plank position.

3. Lift your hips upward and extend your legs outward laterally.

4. Lower your hips and bring your legs back to center.

5. Repeat steps 2 through 4 for a set number of repetitions or for a set time.

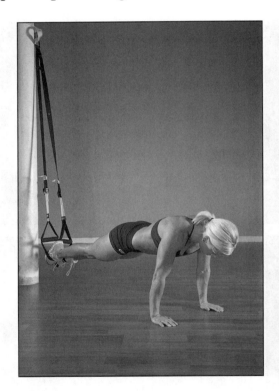
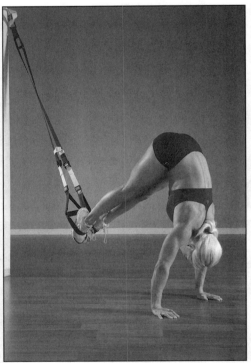

TRX Suspended Side Plank with Twist

1. Lie on your stomach and insert your toes in the TRX toe loops.

2. Turn your body so that you're lying on your side, and prop yourself on the elbow on that side of your body.

3. Raise your hip off the floor, and extend your free arm toward the ceiling.

4. Twist your body toward the floor, and reach your free arm around your body.

    Your goal should be to touch your back.

5. Perform the steps in reverse, return to the side plank position, and then perform the exercise on the other side of your body.

6. Repeat steps 2 through 5 for a set number of repetitions or for a set time.

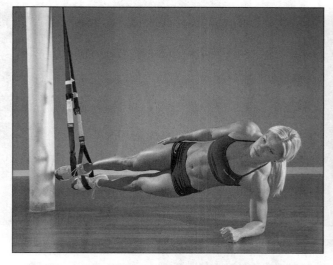
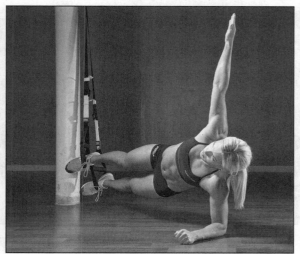
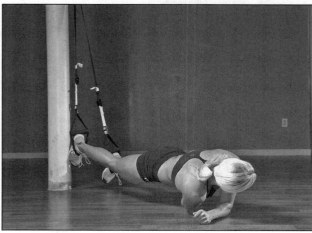
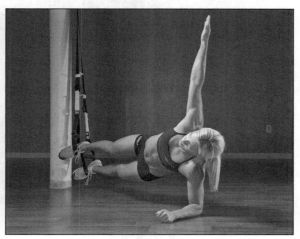

TRX Suspended Side Plank with Twist and Pike

1. Lie on your stomach and insert your toes in the TRX toe loops.

2. Turn your body onto one side and raise yourself up on your elbow.

3. Lift your hip off the floor and extend your free arm toward the ceiling.

4. Twist your body toward the floor and reach your free arm around your body to try to touch your back. While doing so, raise your hips into the air.

5. Lower your hips, rotate in reverse to the start position, and then perform the exercise on the other side of your body.

6. Repeat steps 2 through 5 for a set number of repetitions or for a set time.

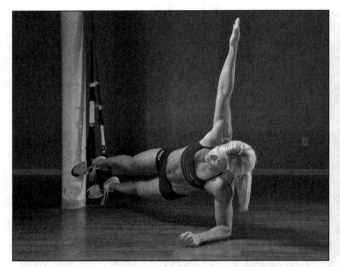
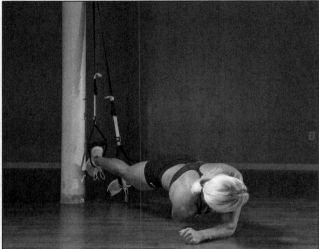
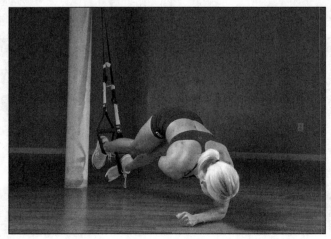

TRX Seated Pull-Up

1. Shorten the TRX straps a little more than usual, so that when you're seated on the floor and reaching up you can just reach the handles.

2. Grasp the handles and sit on the floor with your knees bent.

3. Using primarily your back muscles, pull your body up off the floor.

    Keep your knees bent throughout the exercise. You can use your legs to assist in the upward movement.

4. Lower yourself back down to a seated position.

5. Repeat steps 3 and 4 for a set number of repetitions or for a set time.

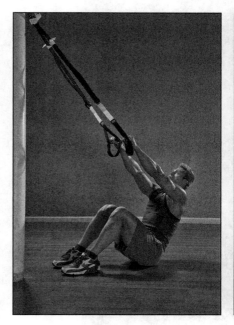
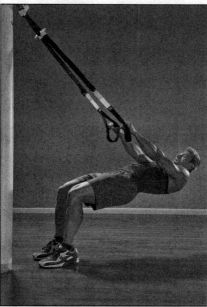
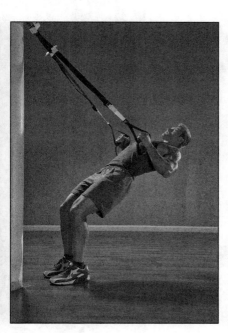

TRX Hack Squat

1. Grasp the handles and extend your arms out in front of you.

2. Holding on to the handles for support, lean back so that you're at least at a 45-degree angle from vertical.

3. Lower your hips by bending your knees while keeping your arms extended.

4. Get your hips as close to the floor as possible and then press your heels into the floor and extend the knees until you return to the start position.

5. Repeat steps 2 through 4 for a set number of repetitions or for a set period of time.

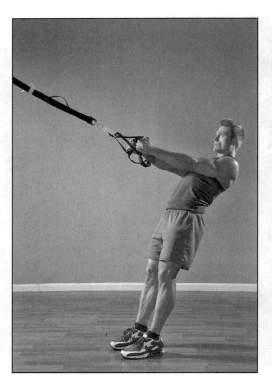
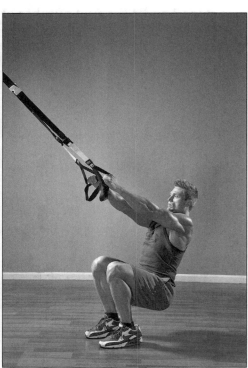

TRX Suspended Walking Planks

1. Lie on your stomach and insert your toes in the TRX toe loops.

2. Raise your body into a push-up plank position.

3. Move your right hand forward and then move your left hand forward.

4. Repeat this "walking" pattern a few more times until you can't go any farther.

5. Reverse the walking pattern until you return to the start position.

6. Repeat steps 2 through 5 for a set number of repetitions or for a set period of time.

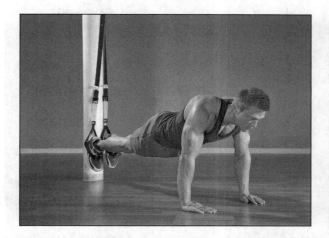
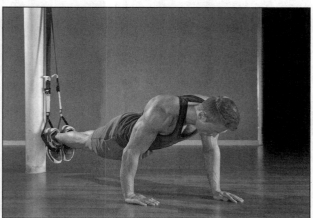
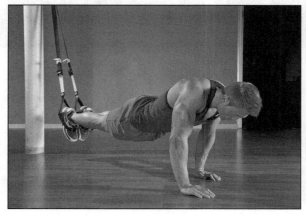
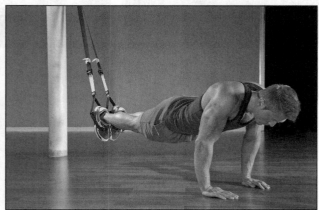

Circle Shoulder Raises

1. Stand holding dumbbells in front of your body with the palms of your hands facing forward.

2. Raise both arms in a semicircle motion over your head until the weights touch over your head.

3. Lower the dumbbells back down to the start position.

4. Repeat steps 2 and 3 for a set number of repetitions or for a set time.

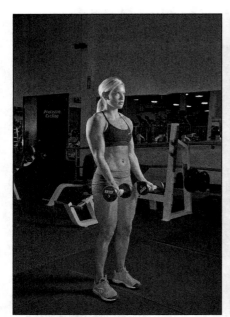 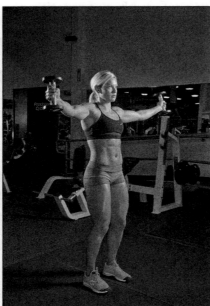 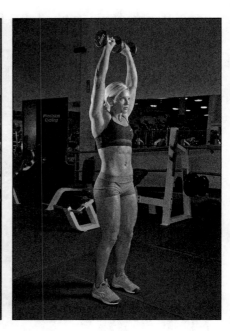

Diagonal Forward Bounding

1. Stand and bend forward at a 45-degree angle.

2. Hop forward and to your right (at a diagonal) so that your right leg lands in a lunge position.

3. Keeping the slight bend at the waist, hop forward and to your left, so that your left leg lands in a lunge position.

4. Repeat steps 2 and 3 for a set number of repetitions or set distance.

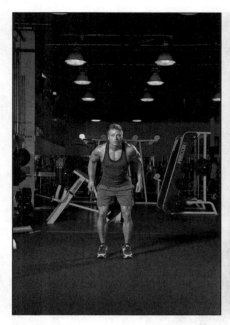
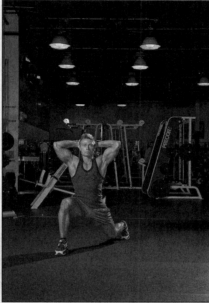
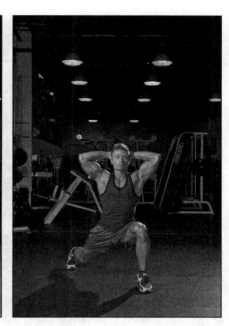

Powerdive Push-Up

1. Lie on your stomach and raise yourself into push-up plank position with your hips lifted high toward the ceiling.

2. Lower your head and chest toward the floor. As your chest gets close to the floor, arch your back as you push your chest upward.

3. Reverse the action and push your hips back and up toward the ceiling to the start position.

4. Repeat steps 2 and 3 for a set number of repetitions or for a set time.

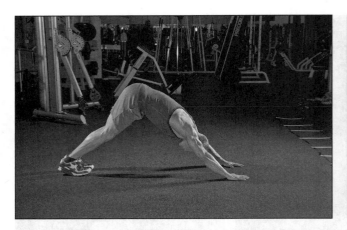
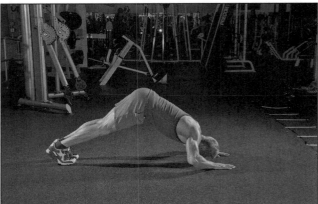
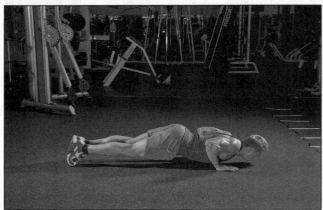
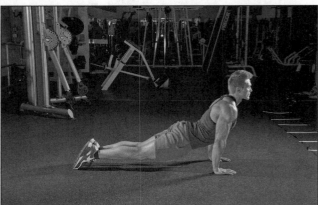

BOSU Balance Trainer High Knees with One Leg On and One Leg Off

1.   Place your right foot on the BOSU and squat down until your left knee touches the floor.

2.   Explode up by pushing down with your right leg and lifting your left knee off the floor.

3.   Land with your left foot on the BOSU and squat down until your right knee touches the floor.

4.   Explode up by pushing down with your left leg and lifting your right knee off the floor.

5.   Repeat steps 2 through 4 as quickly as you can for a set number of repetitions or for a set time.

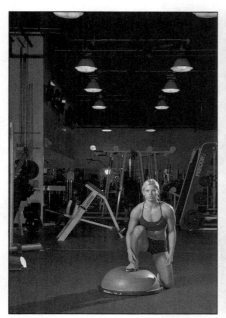 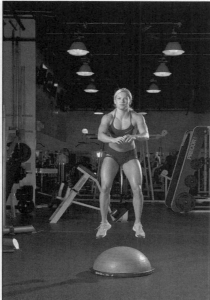 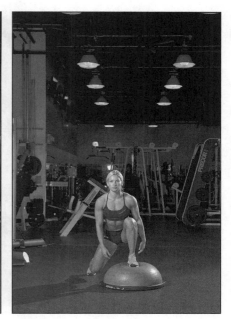

Note

A BOSU Balance Trainer looks like an exercise ball that has been cut in half and attached to a stable base. You can use the BOSU Balance Trainer for a number of exercises that strengthen your core, increase balance, and improve overall strength. When you balance on a BOSU to exercise, you engage stabilizer muscles throughout your body (more than you would if you did the same exercise on a stable surface such as the floor), thereby increasing your overall strength, balance, and fitness.

Forward Hurdle Running

1.   Stand facing the hurdles.

2.   Lift your right knee and step over the first hurdle. Then lift your left knee up and step over the first hurdle, moving your body over the first hurdle.

3.   Repeat leg movement pattern over all the hurdles.

4.   Turn around and repeat steps 2 and 3 going in the opposite direction.

5.   Repeat steps 2 through 4 for a set number of reps or time.

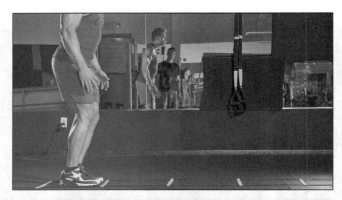

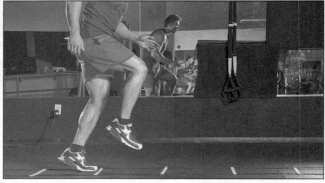

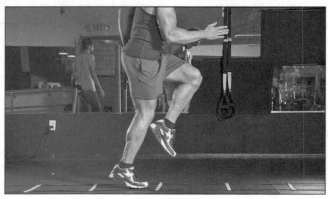

Sideways Hurdle Running

1. **Stand facing sideways to the hurdles.**

2. **Lift your right knee and move your right leg over the first hurdle.**

3. **Lift your left knee, cross your left leg in front of your right leg, and step into the next hurdle.**

    Your body should be over the first hurdle.

4. **Repeat steps 2 and 3 to the end of the hurdles.**

    You can move quickly or slower depending on skill level.

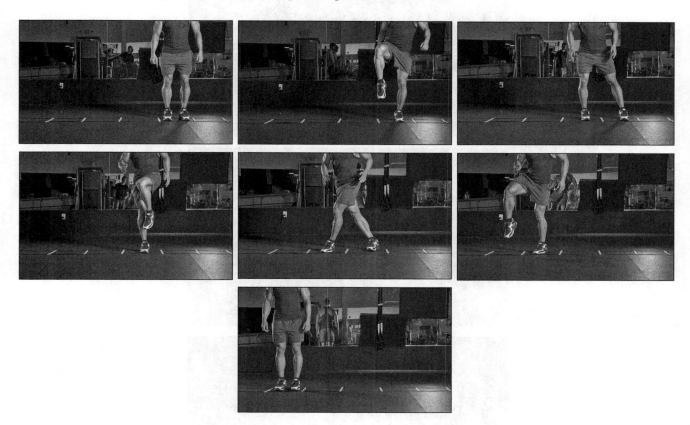

Floor Bear Crawls

1. Start in push-up position or in reverse plank position.

2. Move your left knee forward, and then move your right hand forward.

3. Move your right leg forward, and then move your right hand forward.

4. Repeat steps 2 and 3 for a set distance.

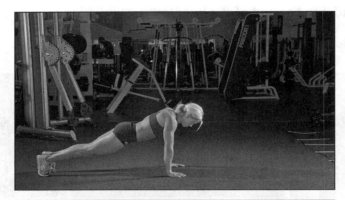

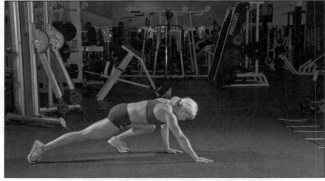

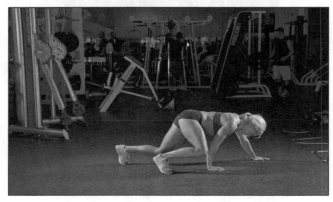

Lateral Box Push-Offs

1. Stand to the side of the box and place your right foot on top of the box.

2. Push off the box using only your right leg and explode vertically as high as possible. Drive your arms forward and up for maximum height.

3. Land with your left foot on the box and right foot on the ground on the other side of the box.

4. Alternating legs, repeat steps 1 through 3 for a set number of repetitions or a set time.

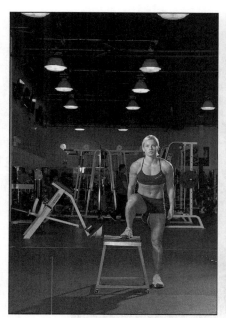 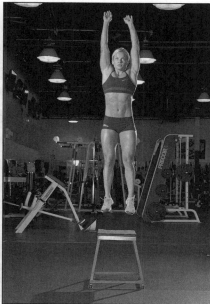 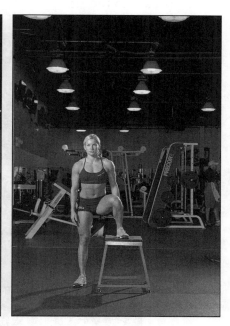

Note

A jump box, also known as a plyometric platform or plyo box, is a sturdy box used for explosive training. Jump boxes come in a variety of heights, and it's best to start out with a lower height and slowly work your way up to higher boxes.

Tuck Jumps

1. **Stand with your feet shoulder-width apart, your knees slightly bent, and your arms at your sides.**

2. **Jump up, bringing your knees up to your chest.**

3. **Land on the balls of your feet, and repeat immediately for a set number of repetitions or a set time.**

   Try to reduce ground contact time by landing softly on the balls of your feet and springing back into the air.

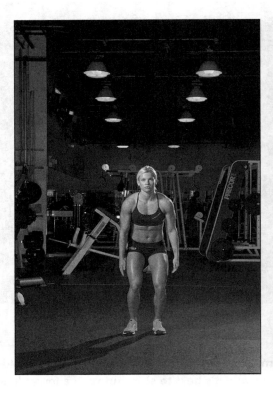 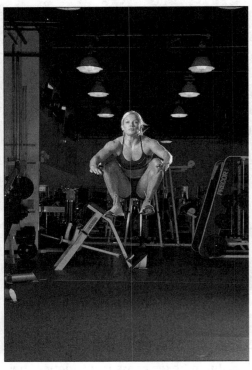

Lateral Hurdle Jumps

1. **Stand beside an object to be cleared.**

2. **Bring your knees up and jump vertically but also laterally off the ground and over the barrier.**

3. **Land on both feet and immediately jump the other direction over the barrier.**

    Try not to pause between jumps or sink down into a squat position.

4. **Repeat steps 2 and 3 for a set number of repetitions or for a set time.**

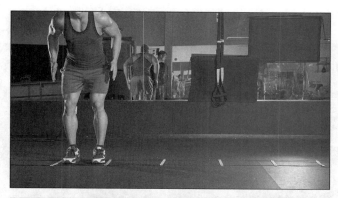

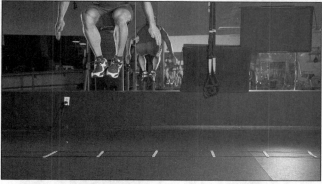

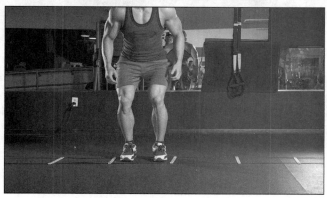

Lateral Jump to Box

1. **Stand beside a box with your feet spread slightly.**

2. **Lower your body into a semisquat position and jump up onto the box.**

   Don't hold the squat position before jumping up; instead, try to keep the time between dipping down and jumping up to a minimum.

   Your feet should land softly on the box.

3. **Step (don't jump) back down on the same side to your start position.**

4. **Repeat steps 2 and 3 for a set number of repetitions for each leg.**

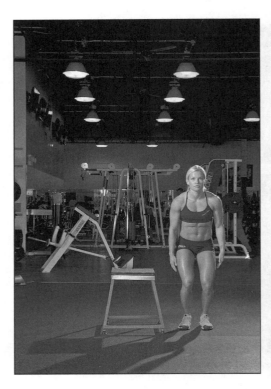 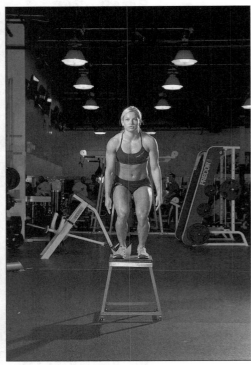

When first starting out using a jump box, focus less on the height of the jump than how you land. Don't hesitate to start out with a very low box—6 to 12 inches is totally fine. When you land, try to do so with a slight bend in your knees and your hips back. Only increase the height of the box when you can maintain proper landing technique.

Explosive Start Throws

1. Stand with your feet slightly wider than hip-width apart.

    Bend your knees slightly.

2. Grasp a medicine ball with both hands and hold it at chest level and close to your body.

3. Explode up with your legs and press the ball straight out as far and as fast as you can, releasing the ball.

4. As you press the ball forward, explode with either leg so that you actually sprint forward a couple of steps.

5. Repeat steps 2 through 4, alternating legs, for a set number of repetitions or for a set time.

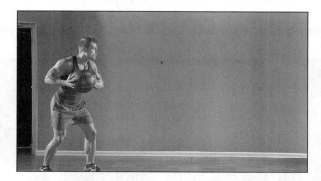

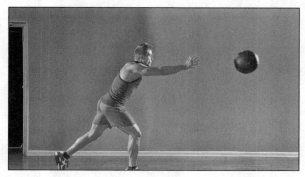

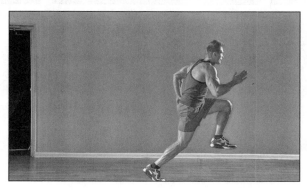

Squat Throws

1. **Holding a medicine ball at chest level and close to your body, stand with your feet slightly wider than hip-width apart.**

    Keep a slight bend in your knees.

2. **Squat down so that your thighs are parallel to the floor.**

3. **Explode up and jump as high as you can. As you start your jump, start to shoulder press the ball up so that your arms are fully extended when you're at the peak of your jump. Push the ball as high as possible into the air.**

    Try to minimize the time spent in the squatted position. It should be a quick squat and jump.

4. **Catch the ball on the bounce and return to start position.**

5. **Repeat steps 2 through 4 for a set number of repetitions or for a set time.**

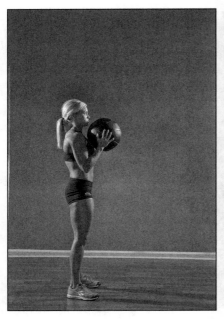 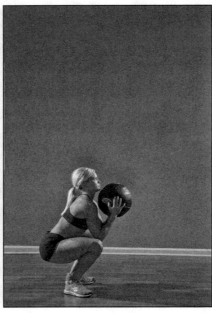 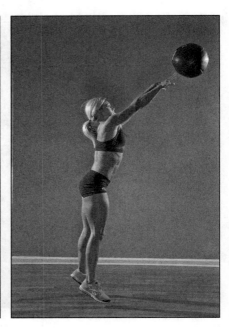

TRX Tornado Twist

1. Grasp the TRX handle with a single hand and face sideways to the anchor. Position the handle and your arms over your head, extend your arms out in front of you, and lean as far back as you can go.

2. Slide your outside leg behind your body and toward the anchor point.

3. Bend the stationary knee to lower your outside hip toward the floor, keeping the back leg straight.

   Your arms will be rotated toward the anchor point as well.

4. While keeping tension on the TRX, push off with the standing leg and engage your core obliques by twisting back up into a standing position.

   You want to bring the outside leg back to the start position.

5. Repeat steps 2 through 4 on the other side.

   Do this exercise for a set number of repetitions or for a set time.

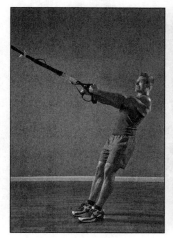
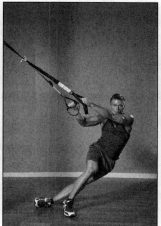
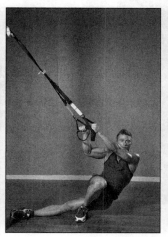
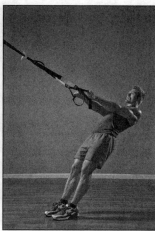

TRX Superman

1. Grasp the TRX handles, face away from the anchor as if you're doing a TRX chest press, bend forward at a 45-degree angle, and extend your arms up like Superman preparing to fly.

2. Lower your hips down and back toward your heels.

    As you bend down, keep your arms extended and swing them out to the side of your body.

3. Push yourself back up to a standing position as you extend your arms back into a Superman position.

4. Repeat steps 2 and 3 for a set number of repetitions or for a set time.

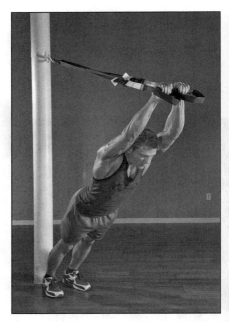
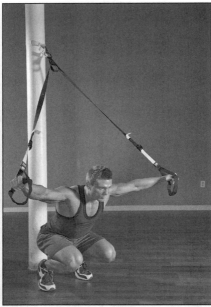
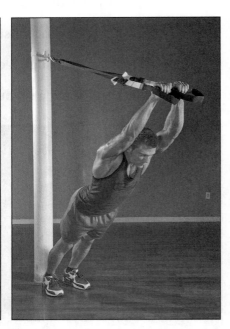

BOSU Reverse Burpee and Roll-Up Squat Hop-Up

1.   Stand facing away from BOSU Balance Trainer.

2.   Lower down and sit on the front edge of BOSU Balance Trainer.

3.   With your arms at your sides, lean back so that you're lying on the BOSU Balance Trainer.

4.   Curl back up to a squat position with your arms reaching out in front of you.

5.   Hop up from the squat position.

6.   Repeat steps 2 through 5 for a set number of repetitions or for a set time.

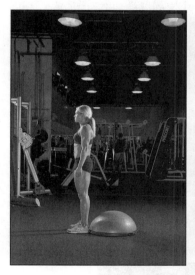
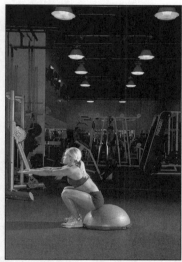
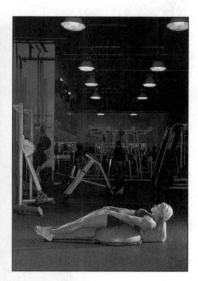

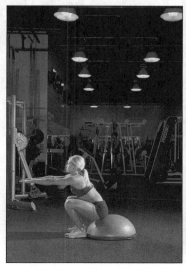
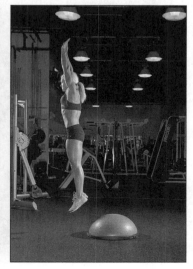

TRX Atomic Push-Ups

1. Lie on your stomach and insert your toes in the TRX toe loops.

2. Raise your upper body into a push-up (keep your hands shoulder-width apart) plank position.

3. Pull both knees in to your chest.

4. Extend your knees back and perform one push-up.

5. Repeat steps 2 through 4 for a set number of repetitions for a set time.

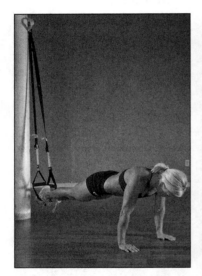
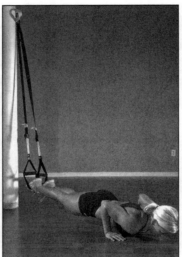
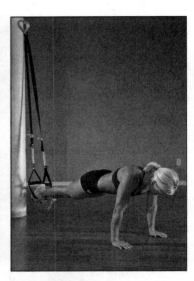

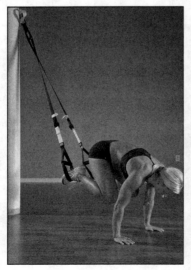
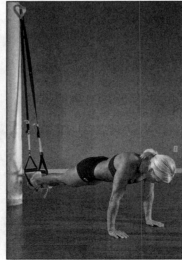

Kneeling to Standing Battling Ropes

1. Kneel on the floor holding a battling rope in each hand.

2. Begin undulating the ropes by raising your arms in an alternating pattern. As you're undulating the ropes, start moving into a standing position by first raising one leg and then the other.

    Continue undulating the ropes throughout this exercise.

3. Lower your body back down to a kneeling position while still undulating the ropes.

4. Repeat steps 2 and 3 for a set number of repetitions or for a set time.

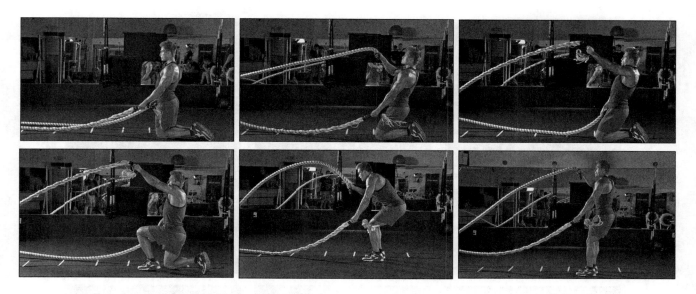

Note

A battling rope is a heavy training rope (1½ to 2 inches thick) you exercise with by swinging your arms up and down or side to side. Rope exercises are a great cardio workout that also strengthens your arms and core.

BOSU Forward Burpee with Squat Hop-Up Onto BOSU

1.   Stand facing a BOSU Balance Trainer.

2.   Squat down and place both palms on top of the BOSU.

3.   Extend both legs behind you by stepping or hopping back.

4.   Step or hop both legs back toward your chest.

5.   Hop up onto the BOSU Balance Trainer.

6.   Repeat steps 2 through 5 for a set number of repetitions or for a set time.

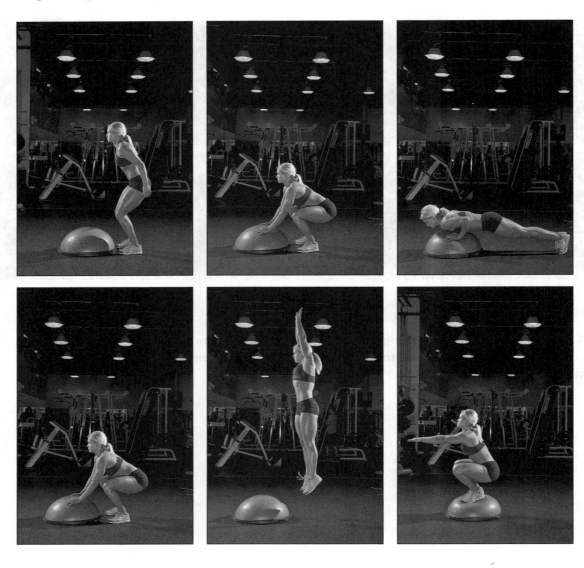

Chapter 8

Core Exercises

Your core includes muscles in your abdomen, lower back, hips, and pelvis. A strong core helps you maintain proper posture and protects your lower back from injury. Certain muscles in the core help keep your waistline looking trim and slim and contribute to fabulous six-pack abs (but your diet plays an even bigger role in your figure).

On the obstacle course, a strong core gives you better overall stability, making it easier to stay upright while slogging through thick sand and mud or knee-deep water. And when you exercise your core, you ensure that the muscles in your abdomen, hips, pelvis, and lower back work together in harmony, which helps you maintain your balance on the log hop and balance beam. Without a strong core, obstacles such as the monkey bars, over-under crawls, and hurdles are going to leave you feeling as limp as last Thursday's leftover lo mein takeout.

Your body may try to compensate for a weak core by relying on your arm and leg muscles to do all the work, but an obstacle course will expose this sham by sapping you of limb strength toward the end of the course, just when you need it most—if only to hoist that well-deserved mug of beer to your lips.

The exercises in this chapter are hardcore workouts for your all-important core.

Floor Oblique Crunch

1. **Lay face up on the floor with your knees bent.**

   Your thighs should be perpendicular to the ground, and your hands should be folded across your chest.

2. **Slowly raise your shoulders up and forward toward your chest, twisting your body to the right.**

   You should feel a contraction in your abdominal muscles.

3. **Reverse direction, returning to the start position.**

   Your abdominal muscles should remain engaged to slowly lower the upper torso back to the start position. Also, by keeping the abs "engaged," you create a stronger mind-to-muscle connection (signal), which will help to recruit more abdominal muscle fibers.

4. **Repeat steps 1 through 3 until you've completed the desired number of repetitions.**

5. **After performing the desired number of repetitions to the right, repeat steps 1 through 4, this time twisting your body to the left.**

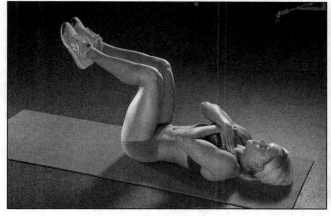 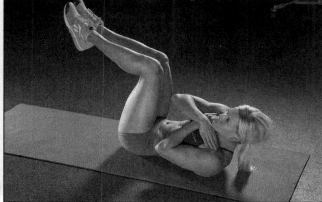

Note

Obliques are actually two sets of muscles—the internal obliques and external obliques—that together make up the sides of your abdomen. Strong obliques protect your lower back from injury and help you rotate your torso and bend sideways. On the obstacle course, strong obliques help you crawl under barbed wire and snake your way through tunnels.

Floor Forward Crunch

1.   **Lay face up on the floor with your knees bent.**

Your thighs should be perpendicular to the ground, and your hands should be folded across your chest or behind your ears. Contract your abdominal muscles before you begin the crunch, and focus your concentration on that contraction.

2.   **Slowly raise your shoulders and chest up and forward without bending your head or neck.**

Exhale as you raise yourself up.

3.   **At the top position, contract your abs hard and hold for two seconds. Return to the starting position using a controlled descent.**

4.   **Repeat steps 2 and 3 for a set number of repetitions.**

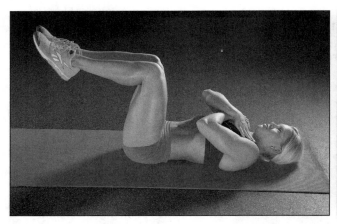 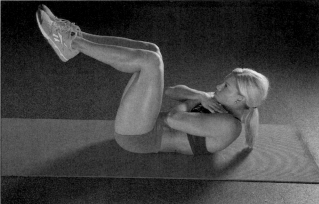

Tip

I see a lot of people race through their crunches as if they're being timed. Although rapid crunches might get you to the showers more quickly, they aren't going to get you to the finish line any faster. Instead of quick movements, raise and lower your chest slowly and steadily. The slower, controlled movement will mean that the muscles are doing the work and not momentum. You build more strength this way, and your core will thank you.

Floor Reverse Crunch

1. **Lay face up on the floor with your knees bent and your thighs perpendicular to the floor.**

    Your lower legs should be horizontal to the floor, and your arms should be down at your sides with your palms flat on the floor.

2. **Curl your hips and pelvis up and back toward your chest.**

    Avoid using momentum to perform the exercise, instead letting your abdominal muscles do the work. At full contraction, squeeze your abs as tight as you can for two seconds.

3. **Slowly return your legs to the start position.**

4. **Repeat steps 2 and 3 for a set number of repetitions.**

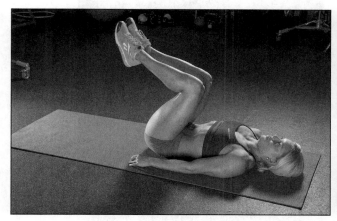 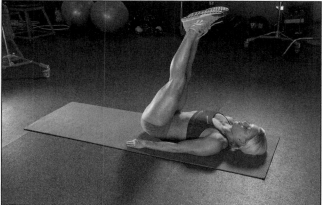

Obstacle Ahead!

Don't try to do this motion quickly; doing so might overstress your lower back and possibly injure it. Focus on contracting your abdominal muscles and pressing your lower back to the ground.

Stability Ball Forward Crunch

1. **Position your lower back on the ball with both feet on the floor.**

   Take a few seconds to find the proper positioning so that you're balanced on the ball.

2. **Place your hands behind your head to support your neck and then inhale to prepare for the exercise.**

3. **Exhale, contract your abdominal muscles, and raise your shoulders forward up off the ball.**

4. **Slowly inhale and reverse direction to the start position.**

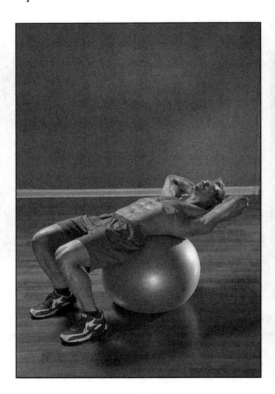 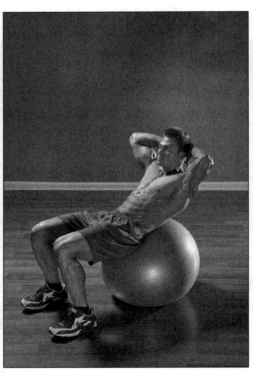

Tip

Try to keep your elbows back and relaxed and your neck in a neutral position while doing crunches on the stability ball. Also, think about moving *upward* rather than forward on your crunches.

Stability Ball Praying Mantis

1. **Stand facing a stability ball, lean forward, and place your forearms on top of the ball.**

2. **Step both feet back until your body is in a plank position.**

    Keep one leg closer to the ball if you can't keep your balance with both legs back.

3. **Hold the plank position for 15, 30, 45, or 60 seconds.**

    Be sure to breathe normally while holding the plank.

4. **Slowly raise yourself back up to standing position.**

5. **Repeat exercise for a set period of time.**

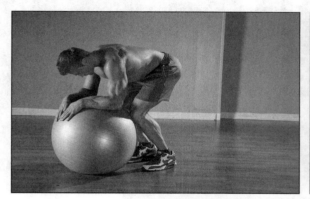
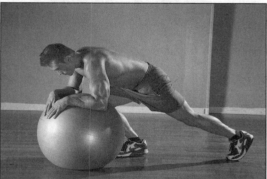
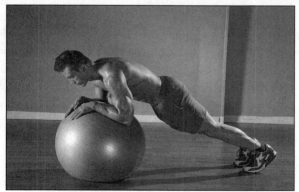

Note

A stability ball, also sometimes referred to as a *Swiss ball,* is a large, inflatable, plastic ball used in many exercise programs. Because you have to work to maintain balance while exercising on the ball, you engage more muscles than you would if you did the same exercise on a static surface. If you use the ball consistently, you will develop stronger muscles. Your gym should have stability balls, or you can purchase your own at big-box department stores such as Target, Sears, or Kmart.

Floor Push-Up Plank

1. Lie on your stomach with your palms on the floor under your shoulders, your feet together, and your spine in a neutral position.

2. Lift your body up on your palms and toes, keeping your head, torso, and legs in a straight line.

3. Maintain this position for at least a minute.

    Challenge yourself to maintain the plank position for 10 seconds longer each time you perform it.

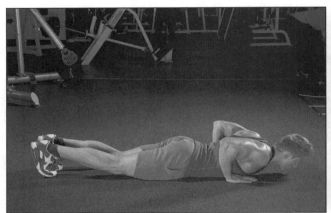 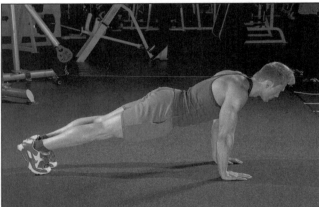

Tip

Planks are static exercises, meaning they don't involve any movement. After you assume the correct position, you should be still for the duration of the exercise. An exercise without any movement might sound like cheating, but when done properly, static exercises can make for a very rigorous workout. Holding a static contraction means you are stabilizing the core and simultaneously working on strength and muscular endurance within the entire core. Overloading the lower back with *only* crunches or sit-ups can put way too much pressure on the spinal column, especially the lower-back region.

TRX Side Elbow Plank

1. **Lay on your left side and place your feet in the TRX straps, your left elbow on the floor, and your shoulders over your elbow.**

    Make sure your feet are stacked on top of each other.

2. **Raise your left hip off the floor, keeping it in line with your shoulder, and then place your free hand on your right hip or raise it up toward the ceiling.**

    Hold this position for as long as possible.

3. **Repeat steps 1 and 2 on the opposite side.**

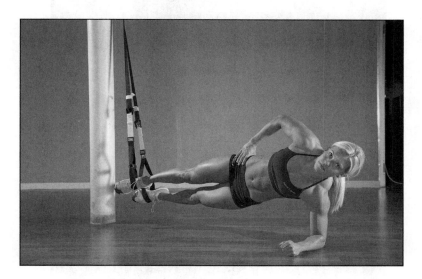

Floor V Crunch (Single Leg)

1. Lay face up on the floor with your legs straight out and your arms extended out in front of you.

2. Lift your right leg from the hip into the air; when it's about 45 degrees off the floor, crunch your chest forward toward your ankle.

3. Lower your leg and upper body to the floor.

4. Repeat steps 1 through 3 with your left leg.

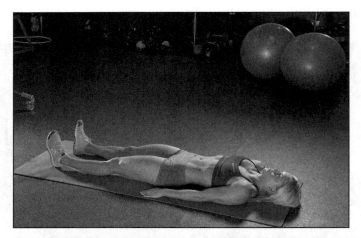

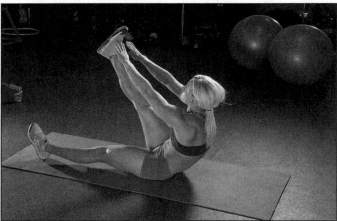

Note

Crunches help strengthen your rectus abdominus muscle, which runs the entire length of your abdomen and is the muscle responsible for six-pack abs. Think of your six pack as buried treasure. Most people have a lot more abdominal muscle than they are aware of. They don't know it, because they can't see or perhaps can't even feel it. Your job is to excavate through the fat, via exercise and diet, to reveal the abs.

Floor Pendulum Oblique Twists

1. **Lay face up on the floor with your knees bent at 90 degrees so your shins are parallel to the floor.**

2. **Drop both knees down to one side, keeping your knees at 90 degrees.**

   Touch your bottom knee down to the ground if possible.

3. **Raise both knees back to start position.**

4. **Repeat exercise on the other side of the body.**

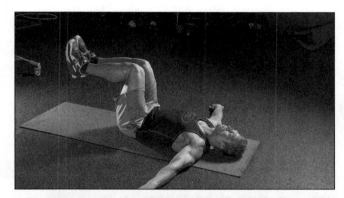

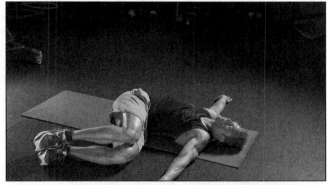

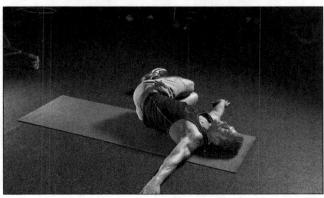

Chapter 9

Cardio Exercises

Attention couch potatoes: I have some good news and some bad news when it comes to cardio training for obstacle races. If you're the kind of person who likes to get the good news first, skip a couple of paragraphs until you see the italic font heralding happier times. If you're like me and prefer to get the negative stuff out of the way first, just keep reading ….

You can probably file this under the "stuff I already knew" category, but if you haven't done much running, biking, swimming, or other aerobic activity lately, the first week or two of cardio training isn't going to be much fun. You're going to be out of breath quickly, you're going to want to stop almost immediately, and you might even feel a lot of jiggling in places that never used to jiggle. I would bet big chunks of my paycheck that you're going to start thinking that maybe this whole train-for-an-obstacle-race business is a silly idea.

Fortunately, it won't take you long to start recognizing *the good news:* after a week or two of steady training, you'll begin to build endurance and lung capacity that you may not have had since you were a kid. Workouts will no longer feel like a steady progression through Dante's nine circles of hell. And you will even begin to enjoy yourself. That's because with every heart-thumping mountain climber, burpee, and jumping jack you're building endurance, which is merely the capacity to withstand the stress of exertion.

If you have to pare down your obstacle race training to the absolute minimum, cardio training should be the last thing to go. If you think of an obstacle race as a pie, the running component comprises the biggest single slice of that pie, so cardio must be the biggest part of your training. And running successfully is more about your cardio fitness level than anything else. (Lower-body strength plays a key role, too; see Chapter 5 to find out how to get a leg up on beefing up those lower-body muscles.)

And keep this in mind, too: you can have the most fab abs and chiseled chest on the course, but if you don't have a strong heart and lungs to back them up, you'll be so far behind the rest of the pack that nobody will even notice your six pack.

Jumping Jacks

1.   Stand with your arms down at your side.

2.   Raise your arms over your head as you hop up and land with your legs apart.

3.   Immediately lower your arms back down as you hop back to a standing position.

4.   Repeat continuously for a set number of reps or period of time.

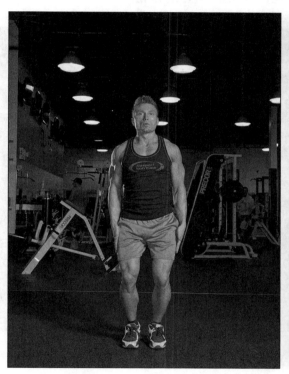
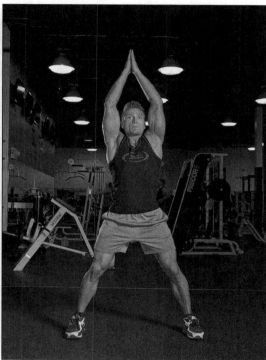

High Knees in Place

1. **Stand with your arms at your sides and your elbows bent at 90 degrees.**

2. **Raise your right knee as high as possible while simultaneously raising your left arm.**

    Your arm and leg movements follow a jogging pattern, but for this exercise you don't move forward.

3. **Lower your right knee/left arm and lift your left knee/right arm.**

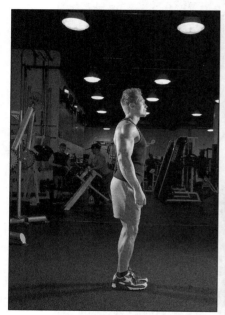 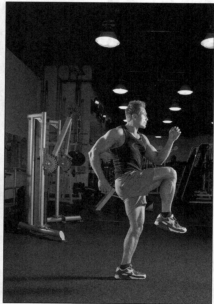 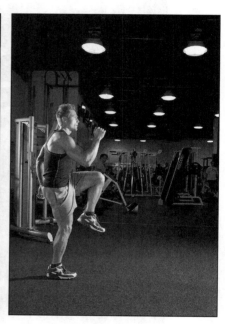

Note

Multiple-time Spartan Race champion Hobie Call doesn't have a bodybuilder's physique, but he does have very strong legs (he holds the world record for fastest lunging mile) and a highly developed cardiovascular system. It's his cardio strength that propels him to the front of the pack.

Jump Rope

1. **Stand holding a jump rope handle in each hand with the rope on the floor behind you.**

2. **Swing the jump rope up and over your head using wrist action and jump over the rope as it comes toward your feet.**

   If you haven't jump roped in a while, you may need some practice to coordinate the timing of the swinging and jumping. Start out at a moderate pace and be patient with yourself.

3. **Continue swinging the jump rope and jumping over rope.**

4. **Repeat for a set number of repetitions or for a set time.**

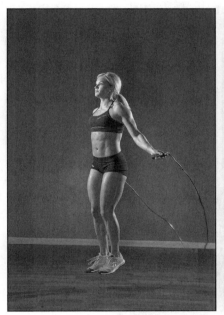
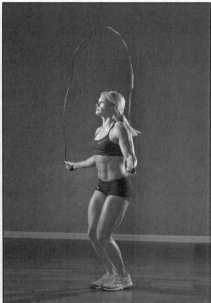
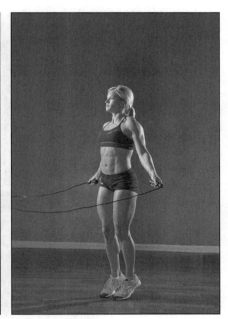

Burpees

1. Stand with your arms hanging down at your sides.

2. Squat down and put your palms on the floor.

3. Extend both legs back into a plank position.

4. Bring both feet in together and under your body, and stand back up with a squatlike movement.

5. Hop up into the air while raising your arms above your head and land in a standing position.

6. Repeat steps 1 through 5 in rapid succession for a set number of repetitions or a set time.

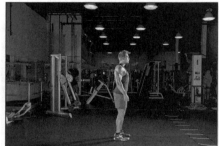 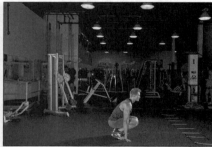 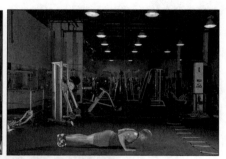

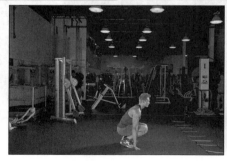 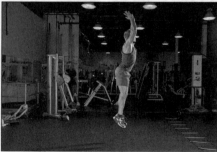

Tip

Running and lunges tend to cause your lower back to get stiff, and burpees are a great way to stretch your lower back. Obstacle race champions throw them in during training runs or other intense cardio workouts to keep the lower back loose without taking a rest.

Mountain Climbers

1. Begin in the push-up plank position, resting your weight on your palms (with arms straight) and your toes.

2. Bring one knee in toward your chest and then extend the knee back to the start position.

3. Bring your other knee in toward your chest and then extend the knee back to the start position.

4. Alternate steps 2 and 3.

5. Repeat for set number of repetitions or for a set time.

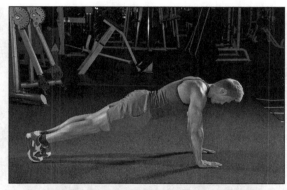

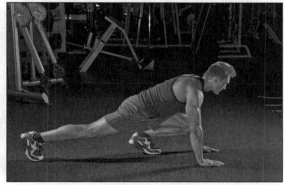

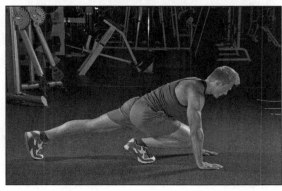

Power Jacks

1. Squat with your arms at your side.

2. Hop up and spread your legs laterally as you raise your arms over your head.

    This is similar to a jumping jack motion.

3. Lower your arms and return to the squat position.

4. Repeat steps 2 and 3.

5. Repeat for a set number of repetitions or for a set time.

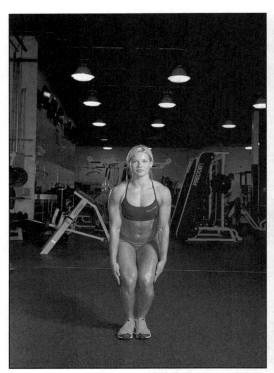
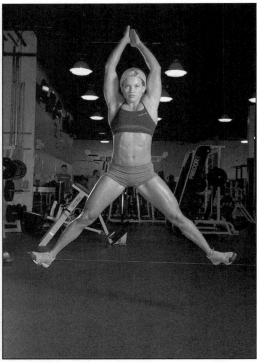

Plank Lateral Jacks

1. Begin in the push-up plank position, resting your weight on your palms (with arms straight) and your toes.

2. Holding the plank, move your right leg laterally away from center position, keeping it lifted off the floor the entire time.

3. Bring your right leg back toward center position.

4. Repeat steps 2 and 3 with your left leg.

5. Repeat exercise for a set number of repetitions or for a set time.

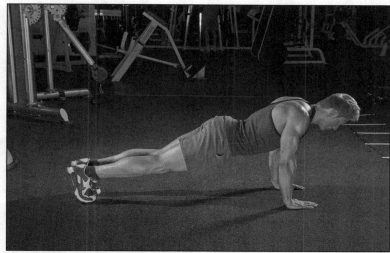

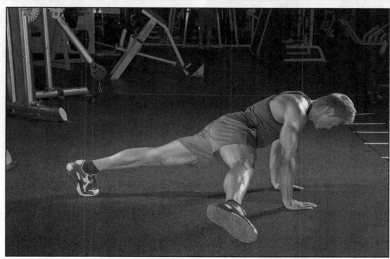

Plank Double Leg Lateral Hops

1. Begin in the push-up plank position, resting your weight on your palms (with arms straight) and your toes.

2. With both legs, hop to your right side.

3. With both legs, hop to your left side.

4. Return both legs to center.

5. Repeat exercise for a set number of repetitions or for a set time.

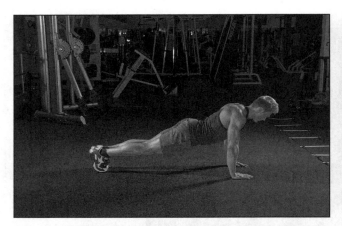
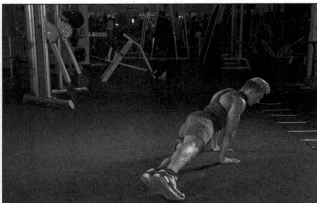
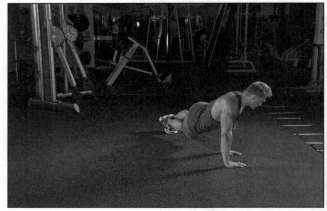
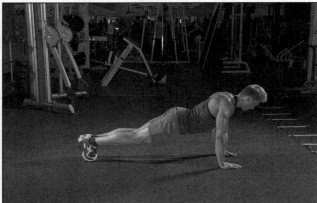

Forward and Backward Jumping

1. Stand with your arms at your side facing a line in the floor.

2. With both feet, jump over the line and then jump back to your start position.

3. Repeat exercise for a set number of repetitions or for a set time.

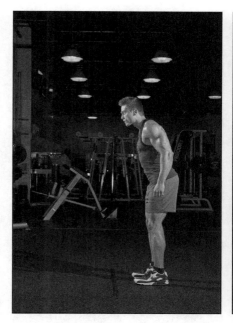
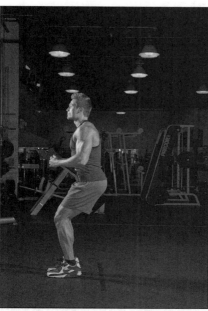
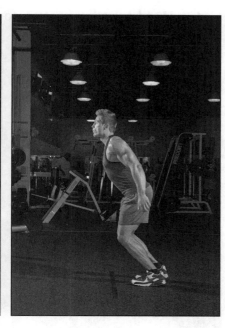

Lateral Jumping

1. Stand with your feet shoulder-width apart.

2. Lower down into the squat position and then hop up and laterally.

3. Continue hopping movements for a set number of repetitions or for a set distance.

4. Hop back to your start position.

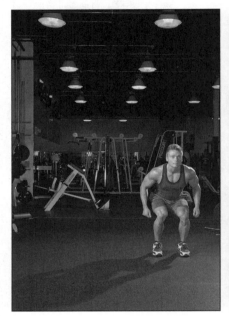
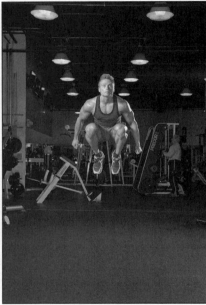
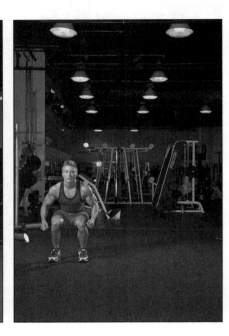

Chapter 10

Race Flexibility

Flexibility is key to avoiding injury on the obstacle course. Although there's no surefire way to protect yourself from muscle strains and tears or tendon, joint, and ligament damage, maintaining limber limbs and muscles can minimize the risks. That's because when you're flexible, your body is better prepared to take the abuse of the obstacle course.

If you slip on a muddy hillside or land awkwardly as you leap a fire obstacle or mud pit, you're less likely to pull your hamstring or calf if those muscles are used to getting a good stretch. Similarly, obstacles such as monkey bars, rope climbs, and spear throws are less of a risk for leaving you with a torn rotator cuff, pulled oblique, or strained bicep if you have full range of motion on those body parts and they're loose, limber, and ready for action. Even simple ankle and shoulder rotations prior to a race can minimize the effects of a turned ankle or strained rotator cuff.

Hamstring Stretch

1.   Sit on the floor with your legs extended forward.

2.   Bend your left knee inward toward the other leg while keeping your right leg straight.

3.   Lean forward as far as you can, and reach toward your right foot.

     Hold this position for 10 to 20 seconds on each repetition.

4.   Repeat steps 2 and 3 with the other leg.

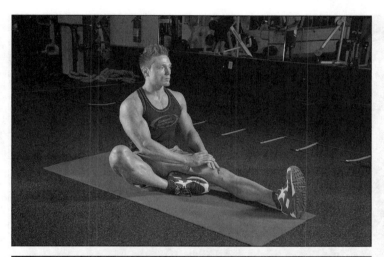

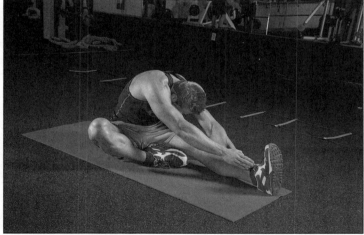

Quadriceps Stretch

1.   Sit on the floor with one leg straight and one leg bent back toward your glutes.

2.   Slowly lean back toward the floor.

3.   Lay back as far as you can, trying to touch your shoulders to the floor.

     Hold this position for 10 to 20 seconds on each repetition.

4.   Repeat steps 2 and 3 on the other side.

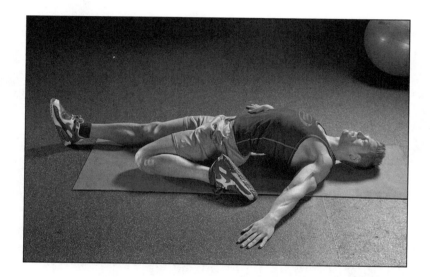

Butterfly Groin Stretch

1. **Sit on the floor and bring the soles of your feet together.**

    Try to maintain a straight spine.

2. **Keeping your back as straight as possible, lean forward and press gently downward on your knees.**

    Hold this position for 10 to 20 seconds on each repetition.

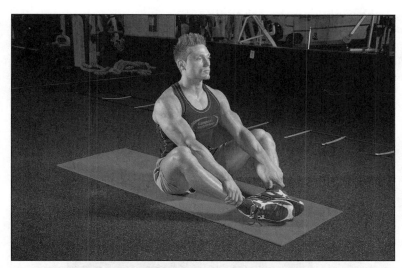

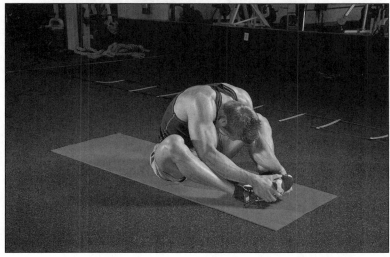

Calf Stretch

1.   Stand with your hands against a wall or a sturdy object.

2.   Step back in a lunge stance.

3.   Bend your front knee until you feel your calf stretch.

     Be sure to keep your back heel down during the stretch. Hold this position for 10 to 20 seconds on each repetition.

4.   Repeat steps 1 through 3 on the other side.

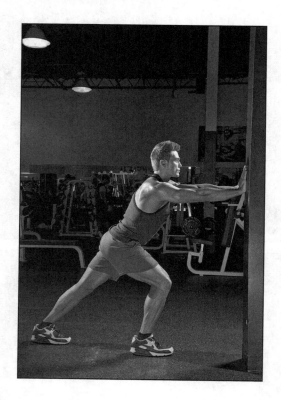

Arm Crossover Shoulder Stretch

1. While standing, bring one arm across your body.

2. With your other hand, press the elbow of the arm across your body into your body.

   Hold this position for 10 to 20 seconds on each repetition.

3. Repeat steps 1 and 2 with your other arm.

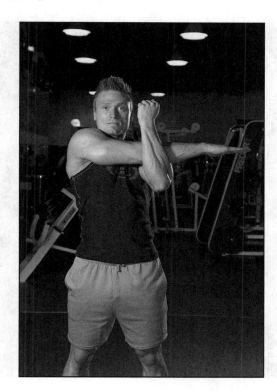

Arm Reach Side Bend Stretch

1.   **Stand with your feet wider than shoulder-width apart.**

2.   **Reach your right arm up toward the ceiling and start leaning to the left.**

       Hold this position for 10 to 20 seconds on each repetition.

3.   **Repeat steps 1 and 2 on the other side.**

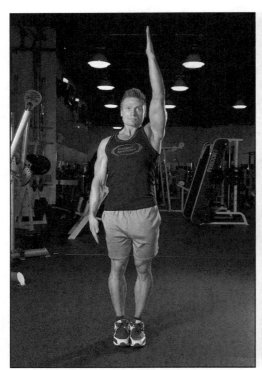 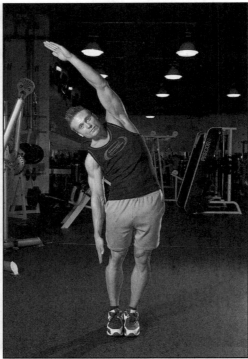

Chest Stretch

1. **Extend one arm out to the side and place it against a wall while keeping your torso parallel to the wall.**

2. **Rotate your opposite shoulder back and gently lean your body against the wall to feel the stretch in your chest and arm.**

    Hold this position for 10 to 20 seconds on each repetition.

3. **Repeat steps 1 and 2 on the other side.**

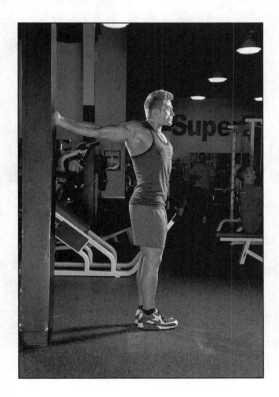

Forward Lean Wide-Stance Back Stretch

1.   **Stand with your feet slightly wider than shoulder-width apart.**

2.   **Bend at the waist and lean forward toward the floor.**

    While keeping your spine straight, try to touch your fingers or even palms to the ground.

    Hold this position for 10 to 20 seconds on each repetition.

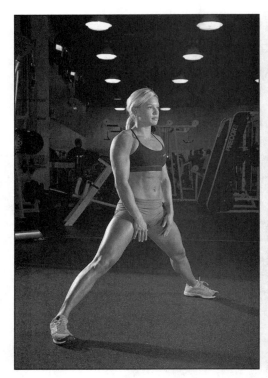 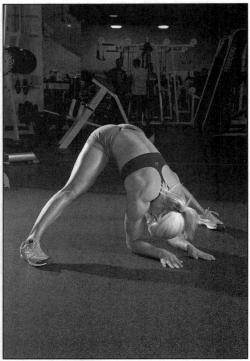

Forearm/Biceps Stretch

1.   Stand with your right arm extended and your fingers pointed down.

2.   With your left hand, pull the fingers of your right hand back until you feel a good stretch.

Hold this position for 10 to 20 seconds on each repetition.

3.   Repeat steps 1 and 2 with the other arm.

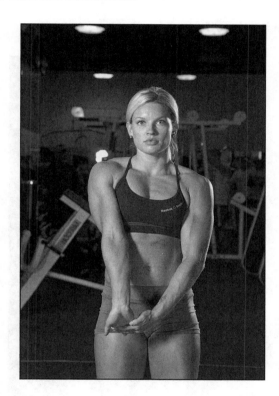

Triceps Stretch

1.   **Stand with your right arm bent at the elbow and above your head so that your right palm is by your right shoulder.**

2.   **Grasp the outside of your right elbow with your left hand and gently press your elbow, moving your right palm down your shoulder blade.**

     Hold this position for 10 to 20 seconds on each repetition.

3.   **Repeat steps 1 and 2 with the other arm.**

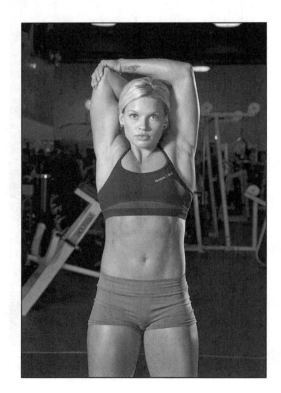

Neck Circles

1. **Stand tall and circle your neck clockwise and then counterclockwise.**

    Several circles in each direction should be enough to loosen up your neck muscles.

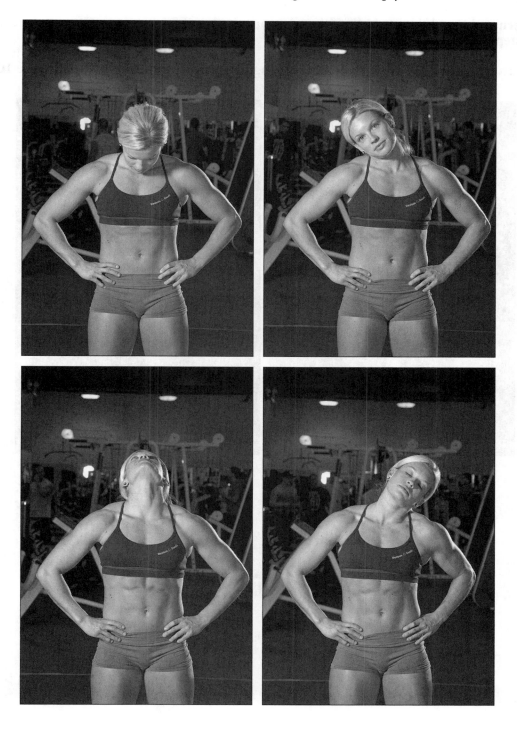

Walking Straight Leg Kick

1. Stand tall and kick your right leg up toward the ceiling.

2. As you kick, reach your left hand toward your right toe.

3. Alternate legs while reaching with your opposite hand for your toe as you "walk" forward 10 steps.

4. Alternate legs as you walk back (continuing to reach with the opposite arm) the 10 steps.

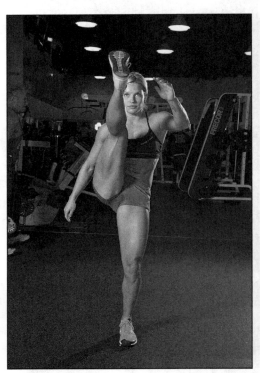
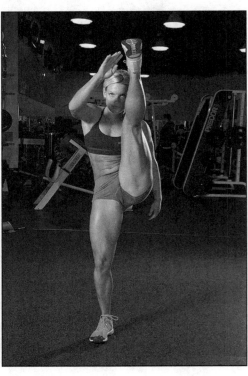

Swimmers Arm Circles

1. Stand tall with your hands hanging to the side of your body.

2. Circle both arms in a forward motion for 10 repetitions.

3. Circle both arms in a backward motion for 10 repetitions.

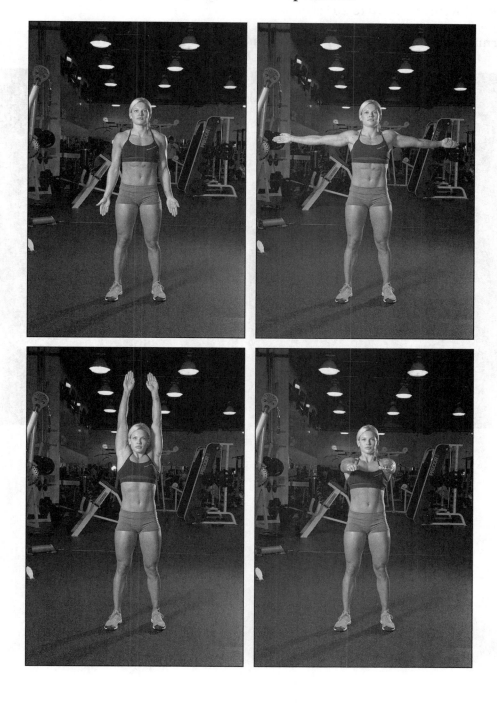

Arm Crosses

1. Stand with your feet shoulder-width apart.

2. Keeping your elbows straight, swing your arms across your body so that your elbows touch where your arms cross.

   Repeat movement for 10 to 20 seconds.

3. Alternate arms so that the opposite arm is on top every other swing.

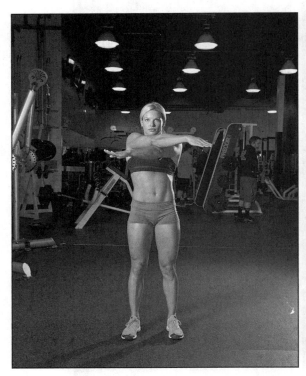
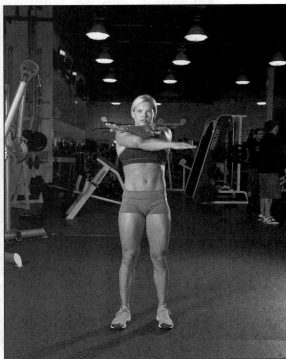

Chapter 11

The Eight-Week Obstacle Race Workout

Part of the fun of preparing for an obstacle race is studying the obstacles and deciding on a plan of attack. You can find plenty of tips for tackling most of the obstacles and challenges you'll encounter in an obstacle race in Chapter 3. However, if you don't have the strength or cardiovascular endurance to execute those tactics, all that planning is for naught. That's where this chapter comes in: an eight-week total body workout program for beginner, intermediate, and advanced athletes looking to conquer any obstacle course race.

This obstacle race training program gives competitors of all fitness levels a guide and workout system to become more fit and healthier for any physical challenge. A training program is intended to maximize the benefits of exercises by putting them in combinations that increase strength and conditioning. Although you can certainly do random sequences of the exercises outlined in Chapters 5 through 9, you get a lot more out of them if you follow a training program.

About Obstacle Race–Specific Training

The training program featured in this book is designed around periodization training, which is just a fancy way of saying that you never overwork any particular group of muscles. Instead, the program devotes a certain percentage of each workout to specific muscle groups and a specific training outcome. The program focuses on three training outcomes:

- **Neurological adaptation/muscular endurance:** This program helps you develop stronger, more efficient connections between your brain and your muscle cells. In turn, the muscle cells learn to use oxygen more efficiently.
- **Strength:** Strength is the ability to exert force on objects using muscles. Physical strength is measured with resistance. For example, your ability to chest press a loaded barbell represents muscular strength.
- **Power:** Power is the amount of force that is exerted during an explosive maximum muscular contraction. You see power demonstrated when someone performs a movement or exercise in a quick and explosive act.

Each week's workout emphasizes different training outcomes. A sample week's workout emphasis might look something like this:

- 50 percent focus on developing neurological adaptation/muscular endurance
- 30 percent focus on strength
- 20 percent focus on power

The second week, the emphasis might shift to strength, as follows:

- 50 percent focus on strength
- 30 percent focus on power
- 20 percent focus on neurological adaptation/muscular endurance

This particular cycle is designed to "wake up" your neurological system to ensure that you're primed and ready for the more advanced stages of your training. Easing into your training reduces the likelihood of burnout and minimizes the chance of injuring your joints, muscles, and connective tissue.

As you begin your training, your mind-to-muscle connection will become enhanced, your exercise coordination will greatly improve, and although this is just the beginning of your training, you will absolutely see dramatic results in your body and conditioning.

Before embarking on your obstacle race training program, you need to do a quick fitness assessment to determine which level is most suitable for you.

Assessing Your Fitness Level

To determine which level program (beginner, intermediate, or advanced) to follow, complete the following fitness assessment:

1. How long does it take you to run 1 mile on relatively flat terrain?

More than 15 minutes	1
12–14.59 minutes	2
9–11.59 minutes	3
6–8.59 minutes	4
Less than 5.59 minutes	5

2. How many pull-ups can you do?

   Men:

0–5	1
6–9	2
10+	3

   Women:

0–4	1
5–8	2
9+	3

3. How many push-ups can you do?

   Men:

0–12	1
13–24	2
25+	3

   Women:

0–9	1
10–21	2
22+	3

4. How many burpees can you do in a minute? (For an illustrated explanation of how to do burpees, head over to Chapter 9.)

   Men:

0–18	1
19–28	2
29+	3

Women:

0–15	1
16–26	2
27+	3

Add your four individual fitness level scores together for your total score: _____

If your total score is …	Use this training level
4–6	Beginner
7–9	Intermediate
10–12	Advanced

How to Use the Training Worksheets

The training worksheets are laid out so that you can see what exercises you need to perform each day and record your progress.

Each day has a set routine, with four exercises for each training style.

The worksheets have spaces for up to six workout sets. The number of sets you do increases the deeper you get into your training.

The space marked *Routine* indicates the type of training for that day. Here's how to interpret each ratio:

- **Work-to-rest ratio:** Perform the exercise for the number of seconds specified on the left side of the slash and then rest for the number of seconds indicated on the right side of the slash. For example, if the work-to-rest ratio is 30/60, exercise for 30 seconds and rest for a minute. As you progress deeper into your training and you build endurance and strength, you will increase the exercise time and decrease the rest time. Record your time and number of reps in the boxes provided.

- **Time-under-tension:** This routine designates the number of reps you do in a set time period. If the ratio is 30 reps in 60 seconds, you should aim to perform 30 repetitions of the exercise in a minute. Record the weight (in LBS) and number of reps in the boxes provided.

Follow these steps to fill in the worksheets:

1. **Fill in the date.**

2. **Perform the routine for the day for each training style.**

3. **Record the pounds (LBS) or Time (TIME) and reps for each set.**

   This helps you track your conditioning progress over the eight-week training period.

4. **Repeat steps 1 through 3 for each training program.**

Endurance Training

If you've already run a number of races at the 5k distance, you probably aren't going to be content to merely finish your obstacle race. You'd like to finish it with grace, in style, and maybe improve your time (known as setting a Personal Record, or PR).

To set a PR, you need to improve your endurance and your speed. You can do this by (1) running more miles, (2) running faster, or (3) performing some combination of both.

> **Note**
>
> **To achieve full benefit from this program, you probably need to have been running three to four days a week for the last year or two, and averaging 15 to 20 miles weekly.**

Here's how to interpret the endurance workout:

- **Run:** When the schedule says to run, aim for an easy pace. How fast is easy? You need to define your own comfort level. Don't worry about how fast you run; just cover the approximate distance suggested. Ideally, you should be able to run at a pace that allows you to converse with a training partner without getting too winded.

- **Fast:** For several of the Saturday runs, I suggest that you run "fast." How fast is "fast"? Again, that depends on your comfort level. Go somewhat faster than you would on a "run" day. If you are doing this workout right, you probably wouldn't be able to carry on a conversation with a training partner. It's okay now to get out of breath.

- **Long Runs:** Once a week, go for a long run. Run 5 to 7 miles at a comfortable pace, not worrying about speed or distance. You should be able to carry on a conversation while you run; if not, you're going to fast. Don't be afraid to stop to walk, or stop to drink. This should be an enjoyable workout, not one during which you punish yourself.

- **Interval Training:** To improve speed, you sometimes need to train at a pace somewhat faster than your race pace for the 5k; run about the pace you would in a 1,500-meter or 1-mile race. Run 400 meters hard and then recover by jogging and/or walking 400 meters. Before starting this workout, warm up by jogging a mile or two, stretching, and doing a few 100-meter sprints. Cool down afterward with a five-minute jog.

- **Tempo Runs:** This is a continuous run with an easy beginning, a buildup in the middle to near 10k race pace, and then ease back and cruise to the finish. A typical tempo run would begin with 5 to 10 minutes easy running, continue with 10 to 15 minutes faster running, and finish with 5 to 10 minutes cooling down. You can't figure out your pace on a watch doing this workout; you need to listen to your body. Tempo runs are very useful for developing anaerobic threshold—essential for fast 5k racing.

- **Rest:** You can't train hard unless you're well rested. The schedule includes two designated days for rest: Mondays and Fridays. The easy 3-mile runs scheduled for Tuesdays and Thursdays are also to help you rest for harder workouts on other days. The final week before the 5k also is a rest week. You want to taper your training so you can be ready for a peak performance on the weekend.

- **Racing:** Some racing is useful in helping you to peak. Consider doing some other races at 5k to 10k distances to test your fitness. The following schedule includes a test 5k race halfway through the program. You could race more frequently (once every two weeks), but too much racing is not a good idea.

The schedule we provide is only a guide. If you want to do long runs on Saturday rather than Sunday, simply flip-flop the days. If you have an important appointment on a day when you have a hard workout planned, do a similar flip-flop with a rest day. It's less important what you do in any one workout than what you do over the full eight weeks leading up to your race.

Dynamic Warm-Up and Postworkout Flexibility

Here's a nightmare scenario for anyone training for an obstacle race: You finally get up the nerve to enter a race, fork over the $100-or-so entrance fee (nonrefundable and nontransferable, of course), and start training like the maniac that you are—or at least always wanted to be. On your third day of training, you gulp down your morning cup of coffee and immediately dive into your lower-body strength exercises. About 30 seconds into your lunges, you feel a sharp pain and hear a snap. Ouch! You just pulled your hamstring and will be out of commission for the next two to six weeks, depending on the severity of your pull.

The best way to avoid this, and similarly frustrating situations, is to ease your body into and out of your workout. You can do this by performing some simple warm-ups prior to your training session, and doing some quick postrace stretching afterward. Spending just five minutes, getting your body ready for more intensive training, can spare you the days (or weeks) of time off needed to recover from a strained or torn muscle, or other injuries.

The good news is that warming up for your training is a snap. Simply follow the basic Dynamic Warm-Up Routine outlined here before *every* training session.

Dynamic warm-up:

- Walking straight leg kicks (1 minute)
- Swimmers arm circles (1 minute)
- Arm crosses (1 minute)
- Walking high knee lifts (1 minute)

Upon completing your workout, plan to spend five or more minutes stretching. Perform each of the following upper- and lower-body stretches for 45 to 60 seconds.

Upper body:

- Triceps stretch
- Forearm/biceps stretch
- Arm reach side bend
- Arm crossover shoulder stretch
- Neck circles

Lower body:

- Hamstring stretch
- Quadriceps stretch
- Butterfly groin stretch
- Calf stretch
- Chest stretch

Beginner

As a beginner, you train in the gym (or at home) three days a week for 60 to 65 minutes (excluding warm-up and endurance training), each day. Each training day focuses on a different area of the body and is broken up as follows:

Day 1—Upper Body:

- Dynamic warm-up (5 minutes)
- Strength training (15 minutes)
- Functional/compound training (15 minutes)
- Cardio training (15 minutes)
- Core training (10 minutes)
- Flexibility (5 minutes)

Day 2—Lower Body:

- Dynamic warm-up (5 minutes)
- Strength training (15 minutes)
- Functional/compound training (15 minutes)
- Cardio training (15 minutes)
- Core training (10 minutes)
- Flexibility (5 minutes)

Day 3—Full Body:

- Dynamic warm-up (5 minutes)
- Strength training (15 minutes)
- Functional/compound training (25 minutes)
- Cardio training (10 minutes)
- Core training (5 minutes)
- Flexibility (5 minutes)

Tip

If you're squeezed for time on any given day, do either the strength or functional/compound training and skip the other. No matter how rushed you are, never skip your warm-up or postworkout stretching.

Week 1

During week one, you perform four sets of each exercise listed on the workout sheet. This first week stresses neurological adaptation/muscular endurance (50 percent of the emphasis) over strength (30 percent) or power (20 percent).

For the first few weeks of training your work-to-rest ratio is fairly lopsided in favor of rest (you lucky dog!). Enjoy your extended breather while you can, because as the weeks go by, you'll work more, and rest less. The long break is meant to ease you into the training by giving you a chance to catch your breath between exercises.

Cardio and Core

Date							Date							Date						
Routine	Work-to-rest ratio: 45/45 sec.						Routine	Work-to-rest ratio: 45/45 sec.						Routine	Work-to-rest ratio: 45/45 sec.					
Exercise	Set 1		Set 2		Set 3		Exercise	Set 1		Set 2		Set 3		Exercise	Set 1		Set 2		Set 3	
	TIME	REPS	TIME	REPS	TIME	REPS		TIME	REPS	TIME	REPS	TIME	REPS		TIME	REPS	TIME	REPS	TIME	REPS
Floor Forward Crunch							Floor Push-Up Plank							Floor Oblique Crunch						
Mountain Climbers							Burpees							Mountain Climbers						
Floor Reverse Crunch							TRX Side Elbow Plank							Stability Ball Forward Crunch						
Jumping Jacks							Lateral Jumping							Jump Rope						
	Set 4		Set 5		Set 6			Set 4		Set 5		Set 6			Set 4		Set 5		Set 6	
	TIME	REPS	TIME	REPS	TIME	REPS		TIME	REPS	TIME	REPS	TIME	REPS		TIME	REPS	TIME	REPS	TIME	REPS
Floor Forward Crunch							Floor Push-Up Plank							Floor Oblique Crunch						
Mountain Climbers							Burpees							Mountain Climbers						
Floor Reverse Crunch							TRX Side Elbow Plank							Stability Ball Forward Crunch						
Jumping Jacks							Lateral Jumping							Jump Rope						

Upper and Lower Body

Date							Date							Date						
Routine	Upper Body Time-under-tension: 15 reps in 60 sec.						Routine	Lower Body Time-under-tension: 15 reps in 60 sec.						Routine	Lower Body Time-under-tension: 15 reps in 60 sec.					
Exercise	Set 1		Set 2		Set 3		Exercise	Set 1		Set 2		Set 3		Exercise	Set 1		Set 2		Set 3	
	LBS	REPS	LBS	REPS	LBS	REPS		LBS	REPS	LBS	REPS	LBS	REPS		LBS	REPS	LBS	REPS	LBS	REPS
Dumbbell Chest Press							Dumbbell Squat							Dumbbell Incline Chest Press						
Dumbbell Chest Flies							Dumbbell Back Lunges							Dumbbell Sumo Squat						
Dumbbell Back Flies							Side Lying Leg Raises							Dumbbell Shoulder Press						
Dumbbell Back Rows							Butt Hip Raises							Dumbbell Incline Biceps Curl						
	Set 4		Set 5		Set 6			Set 4		Set 5		Set 6			Set 4		Set 5		Set 6	
	LBS	REPS	LBS	REPS	LBS	REPS		LBS	REPS	LBS	REPS	LBS	REPS		LBS	REPS	LBS	REPS	LBS	REPS
Dumbbell Chest Press							Dumbbell Squat							Dumbbell Incline Chest Press						
Dumbbell Chest Flies							Dumbbell Back Lunges							Dumbbell Sumo Squat						
Dumbbell Back Flies							Side Lying Leg Raises							Dumbbell Shoulder Press						
Dumbbell Back Rows							Butt Hip Raises							Dumbbell Incline Biceps Curl						

Obstacle Ahead!

If it's been a while since you've worked out, expect to be sore for the first few weeks. Some days you might even feel as though someone pounded your muscles with a meat cleaver. This tenderness is normal! Don't use sore muscles or tired limbs as an excuse for skipping a training session. After a few weeks, your muscles will be used to the training and all you'll notice is your increased energy and strength.

Compound and Functional

Date							Date							Date						
Routine	Work-to-rest ratio: 30/60 sec.						Routine	Work-to-rest ratio: 30/60 sec.						Routine	Work-to-rest ratio: 30/60 sec.					
Exercise	Set 1		Set 2		Set 3		Exercise	Set 1		Set 2		Set 3		Exercise	Set 1		Set 2		Set 3	
	TIME	REPS	TIME	REPS	TIME	REPS		TIME	REPS	TIME	REPS	TIME	REPS		TIME	REPS	TIME	REPS	TIME	REPS
TRX Hack Squat							Forward Hurdle Running							TRX Suspended Leg Circles						
Lateral Box Push-Offs							Sideways Hurdle Running							TRX Suspended V Pike						
Powerdive Push-Up							Floor Bear Crawls							TRX Suspended Side Plank with Twist and Pike						
TRX Seated Pull-Up							Tuck Jumps							TRX Suspended Side Plank with Twist						
	Set 4		Set 5		Set 6			Set 4		Set 5		Set 6			Set 4		Set 5		Set 6	
	TIME	REPS	TIME	REPS	TIME	REPS		TIME	REPS	TIME	REPS	TIME	REPS		TIME	REPS	TIME	REPS	TIME	REPS
TRX Hack Squat							Forward Hurdle Running							TRX Suspended Leg Circles						
Lateral Box Push-Offs							Sideways Hurdle Running							TRX Suspended V Pike						
Powerdive Push-Up							Floor Bear Crawls							TRX Suspended Side Plank with Twist and Pike						
TRX Seated Pull-Up							Tuck Jumps							TRX Suspended Side Plank with Twist						

Endurance

Mon	Tue	Wed	Thu	Fri	Sat	Sun
Rest or run/walk	1.5-mile run	Rest or run/walk	1.5-mile run	Rest	1.5-mile run	30–60 min. walk

Week 2

During week two, continue to do four sets of each exercise listed on the worksheet for that day. The emphasis of these workouts is 50 percent strength, 30 percent power, and 20 percent neurological adaptation/muscular endurance.

Cardio and Core

Table 1

Date						
Routine	Work-to-rest ratio: 45/45 sec.					
Exercise	Set 1		Set 2		Set 3	
	TIME	REPS	TIME	REPS	TIME	REPS
Stability Ball Praying Mantis						
Plank Double Leg Lateral Hops						
Floor Oblique Crunch						
Power Jacks						
	Set 4		Set 5		Set 6	
	TIME	REPS	TIME	REPS	TIME	REPS
Stability Ball Praying Mantis						
Plank Double Leg Lateral Hops						
Floor Oblique Crunch						
Power Jacks						

Table 2

Date						
Routine	Work-to-rest ratio: 45/45 sec.					
Exercise	Set 1		Set 2		Set 3	
	TIME	REPS	TIME	REPS	TIME	REPS
Lateral Jumping						
Floor Push-Up Plank						
Forward and Backward Jumping						
TRX Side Elbow Plank						
	Set 4		Set 5		Set 6	
	TIME	REPS	TIME	REPS	TIME	REPS
Lateral Jumping						
Floor Push-Up Plank						
Forward and Backward Jumping						
TRX Side Elbow Plank						

Table 3

Date						
Routine	Work-to-rest ratio: 45/45 sec.					
Exercise	Set 1		Set 2		Set 3	
	TIME	REPS	TIME	REPS	TIME	REPS
Stability Ball Praying Mantis						
Jump Rope						
Floor Forward Crunch						
Mountain Climbers						
	Set 4		Set 5		Set 6	
	TIME	REPS	TIME	REPS	TIME	REPS
Stability Ball Praying Mantis						
Jump Rope						
Floor Forward Crunch						
Mountain Climbers						

Upper and Lower Body

Table 1

Date						
Routine	Upper Body Work-to-rest ratio: 30/60 sec.					
Exercise	Set 1		Set 2		Set 3	
	LBS	REPS	LBS	REPS	LBS	REPS
Dumbbell Chest Flies						
Dumbbell Biceps Curl						
Pull-Ups						
Chin-Ups						
	Set 4		Set 5		Set 6	
	LBS	REPS	LBS	REPS	LBS	REPS
Dumbbell Chest Flies						
Dumbbell Biceps Curl						
Pull-Ups						
Chin-Ups						

Table 2

Date						
Routine	Lower Body Work-to-rest ratio: 30/60 sec.					
Exercise	Set 1		Set 2		Set 3	
	LBS	REPS	LBS	REPS	LBS	REPS
Dumbbell Pilates Squat						
Dumbbell Calf Raises						
Dumbbell Forward Lunges						
Dumbbell Back Diagonal Lunges						
	Set 4		Set 5		Set 6	
	LBS	REPS	LBS	REPS	LBS	REPS
Dumbbell Pilates Squat						
Dumbbell Calf Raises						
Dumbbell Forward Lunges						
Dumbbell Back Diagonal Lunges						

Table 3

Date						
Routine	Full Body Work-to-rest ratio: 30/60 sec.					
Exercise	Set 1		Set 2		Set 3	
	LBS	REPS	LBS	REPS	LBS	REPS
Chest Dips						
Dumbbell Deltoid Lateral Raise						
Dumbbell Triceps Overhead Extension						
Dumbbell Pilates Squat						
	Set 4		Set 5		Set 6	
	LBS	REPS	LBS	REPS	LBS	REPS
Chest Dips						
Dumbbell Deltoid Lateral Raise						
Dumbbell Triceps Overhead Extension						
Dumbbell Pilates Squat						

Compound and Functional

Date							Date							Date						
Routine	Work-to-rest ratio: 30/60 sec.						Routine	Work-to-rest ratio: 30/60 sec.						Routine	Work-to-rest ratio: 30/60 sec.					
Exercise	Set 1		Set 2		Set 3		Exercise	Set 1		Set 2		Set 3		Exercise	Set 1		Set 2		Set 3	
	TIME	REPS	TIME	REPS	TIME	REPS		TIME	REPS	TIME	REPS	TIME	REPS		TIME	REPS	TIME	REPS	TIME	REPS
Lateral Hurdle Jumps							TRX Atomic Push-Up							Circle Shoulder Raises						
Lateral Jump to Box							BOSU Balance Trainer High Knees with One Leg On and One Leg Off							TRX Seated Pull-Up						
TRX Superman							Explosive Start Throws							TRX Tornado Twist						
Diagonal Forward Bounding							Squat Throws							TRX Atomic Push-Up						
	Set 4		Set 5		Set 6			Set 4		Set 5		Set 6			Set 4		Set 5		Set 6	
	TIME	REPS	TIME	REPS	TIME	REPS		TIME	REPS	TIME	REPS	TIME	REPS		TIME	REPS	TIME	REPS	TIME	REPS
Lateral Hurdle Jumps							TRX Atomic Push-Up							Circle Shoulder Raises						
Lateral Jump to Box							BOSU Balance Trainer High Knees with One Leg On and One Leg Off							TRX Seated Pull-Up						
TRX Superman							Explosive Start Throws							TRX Tornado Twist						
Diagonal Forward Bounding							Squat Throws							TRX Atomic Push-Up						

Endurance

Mon	Tue	Wed	Thu	Fri	Sat	Sun
Rest or run/walk	1.75-mile run	Rest or run/walk	1.5-mile run	Rest	1.75-mile run	30–60 min. walk

Week 3

During week three of training, increase the number of sets from four to five for each exercise prescribed on the worksheets. The breakdown for these workouts is as follows: 50 percent power, 30 percent muscular endurance, 20 percent strength.

Cardio and Core

Date							Date							Date						
Routine	Work-to-rest ratio: 45/45 sec.						Routine	Work-to-rest ratio: 45/45 sec.						Routine	Work-to-rest ratio: 45/45 sec.					
Exercise	Set 1		Set 2		Set 3		Exercise	Set 1		Set 2		Set 3		Exercise	Set 1		Set 2		Set 3	
	TIME	REPS	TIME	REPS	TIME	REPS		TIME	REPS	TIME	REPS	TIME	REPS		TIME	REPS	TIME	REPS	TIME	REPS
Floor Oblique Crunch							Forward and Backward Jumping							Floor Oblique Crunch						
Floor Push-Up Plank							Lateral Jumping							Floor Forward Crunch						
Floor Pendulum Oblique Twists							Burpees							Floor Oblique Crunch						
TRX Side Elbow Plank							Mountain Climbers							Stability Ball Praying Mantis						
	Set 4		Set 5		Set 6			Set 4		Set 5		Set 6			Set 4		Set 5		Set 6	
	TIME	REPS	TIME	REPS	TIME	REPS		TIME	REPS	TIME	REPS	TIME	REPS		TIME	REPS	TIME	REPS	TIME	REPS
Floor Oblique Crunch							Forward and Backward Jumping							Floor Oblique Crunch						
Floor Push-Up Plank							Lateral Jumping							Floor Forward Crunch						
Floor Pendulum Oblique Twists							Burpees							Floor Oblique Crunch						
TRX Side Elbow Plank							Mountain Climbers							Stability Ball Praying Mantis						

Upper and Lower Body

Date							Date							Date						
Routine	Upper Body Time-under-tension: 15 reps in 60 sec.						Routine	Lower Body Time-under-tension: 15 reps in 60 sec.						Routine	Full Body Time-under-tension: 15 reps in 60 sec.					
Exercise	Set 1		Set 2		Set 3		Exercise	Set 1		Set 2		Set 3		Exercise	Set 1		Set 2		Set 3	
	LBS	REPS	LBS	REPS	LBS	REPS		LBS	REPS	LBS	REPS	LBS	REPS		LBS	REPS	LBS	REPS	LBS	REPS
Dumbbell Biceps Curl							Dumbbell Sumo Squat							Dumbbell Chest Flies						
Dumbbell Triceps Kick Back							Dumbbell Calf Raises							Pull-Ups						
Dumbbell Shoulder Press							Dumbbell Back Lunges							Dumbbell Pilates Squat						
Dumbbell Back Flies							Side Lying Leg Raises							Butt Hip Raises						
	Set 4		Set 5		Set 6			Set 4		Set 5		Set 6			Set 4		Set 5		Set 6	
	LBS	REPS	LBS	REPS	LBS	REPS		LBS	REPS	LBS	REPS	LBS	REPS		LBS	REPS	LBS	REPS	LBS	REPS
Dumbbell Biceps Curl							Dumbbell Sumo Squat							Dumbbell Chest Flies						
Dumbbell Triceps Kick Back							Dumbbell Calf Raises							Pull-Ups						
Dumbbell Shoulder Press							Dumbbell Back Lunges							Dumbbell Pilates Squat						
Dumbbell Back Flies							Side Lying Leg Raises							Butt Hip Raises						

Compound and Functional

Date							Date							Date						
Routine	Work-to-rest ratio: 45/45 sec.						Routine	Work-to-rest ratio: 45/45 sec.						Routine	Work-to-rest ratio: 45/45 sec.					
Exercise	Set 1		Set 2		Set 3		Exercise	Set 1		Set 2		Set 3		Exercise	Set 1		Set 2		Set 3	
	TIME	REPS	TIME	REPS	TIME	REPS		TIME	REPS	TIME	REPS	TIME	REPS		TIME	REPS	TIME	REPS	TIME	REPS
TRX Suspended Walking Plank							Lateral Jump to Box							BOSU Forward Burpee with Squat Hop-Up Onto BOSU						
TRX Suspended V Pike							Squat Throws							BOSU Balance Trainer High Knees with One Leg On and One Leg Off						
TRX Superman							TRX Superman							Powerdive Push-Up						
TRX Hack Squat							BOSU Reverse Burpee and Roll-Up Squat Hop-Up							Circle Shoulder Raises						
	Set 4		Set 5		Set 6			Set 4		Set 5		Set 6			Set 4		Set 5		Set 6	
	TIME	REPS	TIME	REPS	TIME	REPS		TIME	REPS	TIME	REPS	TIME	REPS		TIME	REPS	TIME	REPS	TIME	REPS
TRX Suspended Walking Plank							Lateral Jump to Box							BOSU Forward Burpee with Squat Hop-Up Onto BOSU						
TRX Suspended V Pike							Squat Throws							BOSU Balance Trainer High Knees with One Leg On and One Leg Off						
TRX Superman							TRX Superman							Powerdive Push-Up						
TRX Hack Squat							BOSU Reverse Burpee and Roll-Up Squat Hop-Up							Circle Shoulder Raises						

Endurance

Mon	Tue	Wed	Thu	Fri	Sat	Sun
Rest or run/walk	2-mile run	Rest or run/walk	1.5-mile run	Rest	2-mile run	40–60 min. walk

Note

After three weeks of training you should notice a difference in your energy level and maybe even your waistline. Your muscles have gotten used to being worked out, and you are beginning to notice more definition to them.

Week 4

In week four, you continue performing five sets of each exercise. These workouts emphasize 50 percent strength, 30 percent muscular endurance, and 20 percent power.

Cardio and Core

Date						Date						Date					
Routine	Work-to-rest ratio: 45/45 sec.					Routine	Work-to-rest ratio: 45/45 sec.					Routine	Work-to-rest ratio: 45/45 sec.				
Exercise	Set 1		Set 2		Set 3	Exercise	Set 1		Set 2		Set 3	Exercise	Set 1		Set 2		Set 3
	TIME	REPS	TIME	REPS	TIME	REPS		TIME	REPS	TIME	REPS	TIME	REPS		TIME	REPS	TIME	REPS	TIME	REPS
Jumping Jacks							Floor Pendulum Oblique Twists						Plank Lateral Jacks					
Burpees							Floor Oblique Crunch						Forward and Backward Jumping					
Plank Double Leg Lateral Hops							Stability Ball Praying Mantis						High Knees in Place					
Lateral Jumping							Floor V Crunch (Single Leg)						Burpees					
	Set 4		Set 5		Set 6		Set 4		Set 5		Set 6		Set 4		Set 5		Set 6
	TIME	REPS	TIME	REPS	TIME	REPS		TIME	REPS	TIME	REPS	TIME	REPS		TIME	REPS	TIME	REPS	TIME	REPS
Jumping Jacks							Floor Pendulum Oblique Twists						Plank Lateral Jacks					
Burpees							Floor Oblique Crunch						Forward and Backward Jumping					
Plank Double Leg Lateral Hops							Stability Ball Praying Mantis						High Knees in Place					
Lateral Jumping							Floor V Crunch (Single Leg)						Burpees					

Upper and Lower Body

Date						Date						Date					
Routine	Upper Body Work-to-rest ratio: 45/45 sec.					Routine	Lower Body Work-to-rest ratio: 45/45 sec.					Routine	Full Body Work-to-rest ratio: 45/45 sec.				
Exercise	Set 1		Set 2		Set 3	Exercise	Set 1		Set 2		Set 3	Exercise	Set 1		Set 2		Set 3
	LBS	REPS	LBS	REPS	LBS	REPS		LBS	REPS	LBS	REPS	LBS	REPS		LBS	REPS	LBS	REPS	LBS	REPS
Dumbbell Incline Chest Press							Dumbbell Back Lunges						Chin-Ups					
Dumbbell Deltoid Lateral Raise							Dumbbell Squat						Dumbbell Triceps Overhead Extension					
Dumbbell Triceps Skull Crusher							Dumbbell Calf Raises						Chest Dips					
Dumbbell Back Rows							Dumbbell Back Diagonal Lunges						Dumbbell Biceps Curl					
	Set 4		Set 5		Set 6		Set 4		Set 5		Set 6		Set 4		Set 5		Set 6
	LBS	REPS	LBS	REPS	LBS	REPS		LBS	REPS	LBS	REPS	LBS	REPS		LBS	REPS	LBS	REPS	LBS	REPS
Dumbbell Incline Chest Press							Dumbbell Back Lunges						Chin-Ups					
Dumbbell Deltoid Lateral Raise							Dumbbell Squat						Dumbbell Triceps Overhead Extension					
Dumbbell Triceps Skull Crusher							Dumbbell Calf Raises						Chest Dips					
Dumbbell Back Rows							Dumbbell Back Diagonal Lunges						Dumbbell Biceps Curl					

Compound and Functional

Date							Date							Date						
Routine	Work-to-rest ratio: 45/45 sec.						Routine	Work-to-rest ratio: 45/45 sec.						Routine	Work-to-rest ratio: 45/45 sec.					
Exercise	Set 1		Set 2		Set 3		Exercise	Set 1		Set 2		Set 3		Exercise	Set 1		Set 2		Set 3	
	TIME	REPS	TIME	REPS	TIME	REPS		TIME	REPS	TIME	REPS	TIME	REPS		TIME	REPS	TIME	REPS	TIME	REPS
TRX Atomic Push-Up							TRX Suspended Leg Circles							Lateral Box Push-Offs						
Tuck Jumps							TRX Suspended Side Plank with Twist							Lateral Jump to Box						
Squat Throws							Diagonal Forward Bounding							Powerdive Push-Up						
TRX Seated Pull-Up							TRX Atomic Push-Up							BOSU Reverse Burpee and Roll-Up Squat Hop-Up						
	Set 4		Set 5		Set 6			Set 4		Set 5		Set 6			Set 4		Set 5		Set 6	
	TIME	REPS	TIME	REPS	TIME	REPS		TIME	REPS	TIME	REPS	TIME	REPS		TIME	REPS	TIME	REPS	TIME	REPS
TRX Atomic Push-Up							TRX Suspended Leg Circles							Lateral Box Push-Offs						
Tuck Jumps							TRX Suspended Side Plank with Twist							Lateral Jump to Box						
Squat Throws							Diagonal Forward Bounding							Powerdive Push-Up						
TRX Seated Pull-Up							TRX Atomic Push-Up							BOSU Reverse Burpee and Roll-Up Squat Hop-Up						

Endurance

Mon	Tue	Wed	Thu	Fri	Sat	Sun
Rest or run/walk	2.25-mile run	Rest or run/walk	2-mile run	Rest	2.25-mile run	45–60 min. walk

Tip

Now that you've been training for four full weeks, take the Fitness Level Assessment featured earlier in the chapter to check on your progress and see if you should bump up to the next fitness level.

Week 5

From here on out, the workouts have you do six sets of each exercise. Week five's workout focus is 50 percent muscular endurance, 30 percent power, and 20 percent strength.

Cardio and Core

Date						
Routine	Work-to-rest ratio: 60/30 sec.					
Exercise	Set 1		Set 2		Set 3	
	TIME	REPS	TIME	REPS	TIME	REPS
High Knees in Place						
Jump Rope						
Burpees						
Mountain Climbers						
	Set 4		Set 5		Set 6	
	TIME	REPS	TIME	REPS	TIME	REPS
High Knees in Place						
Jump Rope						
Burpees						
Mountain Climbers						

Date						
Routine	Work-to-rest ratio: 60/30 sec.					
Exercise	Set 1		Set 2		Set 3	
	TIME	REPS	TIME	REPS	TIME	REPS
Floor Oblique Crunch						
Stability Ball Praying Mantis						
Floor Pendulum Oblique Twists						
TRX Side Elbow Plank						
	Set 4		Set 5		Set 6	
	TIME	REPS	TIME	REPS	TIME	REPS
Floor Oblique Crunch						
Stability Ball Praying Mantis						
Floor Pendulum Oblique Twists						
TRX Side Elbow Plank						

Date						
Routine	Work-to-rest ratio: 60/30 sec.					
Exercise	Set 1		Set 2		Set 3	
	TIME	REPS	TIME	REPS	TIME	REPS
Floor Forward Crunch						
Lateral Jumping						
Floor Pendulum Oblique Twists						
Plank Double Leg Lateral Hops						
	Set 4		Set 5		Set 6	
	TIME	REPS	TIME	REPS	TIME	REPS
Floor Forward Crunch						
Lateral Jumping						
Floor Pendulum Oblique Twists						
Plank Double Leg Lateral Hops						

Upper and Lower Body

Date						
Routine	Upper Body Time-under-tension: 20 reps in 60 sec.					
Exercise	Set 1		Set 2		Set 3	
	LBS	REPS	LBS	REPS	LBS	REPS
Dumbbell Incline Chest Press						
Dumbbell Triceps Skull Crusher						
Dumbbell Deltoid Lateral Raise						
Dumbbell Back Rows						
	Set 4		Set 5		Set 6	
	LBS	REPS	LBS	REPS	LBS	REPS
Dumbbell Incline Chest Press						
Dumbbell Triceps Skull Crusher						
Dumbbell Deltoid Lateral Raise						
Dumbbell Back Rows						

Date						
Routine	Lower Body Time-under-tension: 20 reps in 60 sec.					
Exercise	Set 1		Set 2		Set 3	
	LBS	REPS	LBS	REPS	LBS	REPS
Dumbbell Squat						
Butt Hip Raises						
Dumbbell Forward Lunges						
Dumbbell Calf Raises						
	Set 4		Set 5		Set 6	
	LBS	REPS	LBS	REPS	LBS	REPS
Dumbbell Squat						
Butt Hip Raises						
Dumbbell Forward Lunges						
Dumbbell Calf Raises						

Date						
Routine	Full Body Time-under-tension: 20 reps in 60 sec.					
Exercise	Set 1		Set 2		Set 3	
	LBS	REPS	LBS	REPS	LBS	REPS
Dumbbell Biceps Curl						
Chest Dips						
Dumbbell Sumo Squat						
Dumbbell Forward Lunges						
	Set 4		Set 5		Set 6	
	LBS	REPS	LBS	REPS	LBS	REPS
Dumbbell Biceps Curl						
Chest Dips						
Dumbbell Sumo Squat						
Dumbbell Forward Lunges						

Compound and Functional

Date							Date							Date						
Routine	Work-to-rest ratio: 60/30 sec.						Routine	Work-to-rest ratio: 60/30 sec.						Routine	Work-to-rest ratio: 60/30 sec.					
Exercise	Set 1		Set 2		Set 3		Exercise	Set 1		Set 2		Set 3		Exercise	Set 1		Set 2		Set 3	
	TIME	REPS	TIME	REPS	TIME	REPS		TIME	REPS	TIME	REPS	TIME	REPS		TIME	REPS	TIME	REPS	TIME	REPS
Forward Hurdle Running							Circle Shoulder Raises							BOSU Balance Trainer High Knees with One Leg On and One Leg Off						
Sideways Hurdle Running							TRX Seated Pull-Up							TRX Suspended Walking Plank						
TRX Tornado Twist							TRX Atomic Push-Up							TRX Suspended Leg Circles						
TRX Superman							BOSU Reverse Burpee and Roll-Up Squat Hop-Up							BOSU Forward Burpee with Squat Hop-Up Onto BOSU						
	Set 4		Set 5		Set 6			Set 4		Set 5		Set 6			Set 4		Set 5		Set 6	
	TIME	REPS	TIME	REPS	TIME	REPS		TIME	REPS	TIME	REPS	TIME	REPS		TIME	REPS	TIME	REPS	TIME	REPS
Forward Hurdle Running							Circle Shoulder Raises							BOSU Balance Trainer High Knees with One Leg On and One Leg Off						
Sideways Hurdle Running							TRX Seated Pull-Up							TRX Suspended Walking Plank						
TRX Tornado Twist							TRX Atomic Push-Up							TRX Suspended Leg Circles						
TRX Superman							BOSU Reverse Burpee and Roll-Up Squat Hop-Up							BOSU Forward Burpee with Squat Hop-Up Onto BOSU						

Endurance

Mon	Tue	Wed	Thu	Fri	Sat	Sun
Rest or run/walk	2.5-mile run	Rest or run/walk	2-mile run	Rest	2.5-mile run	50–60 min. walk

Week 6

During week six, continue performing six sets of each exercise. Your training focus for this week is 50 percent strength, 30 percent power, and 20 percent muscular endurance.

Cardio and Core

Panel 1 — Date: ___ | Routine: Work-to-rest ratio: 60/30 sec.

Exercise	Set 1 TIME	Set 1 REPS	Set 2 TIME	Set 2 REPS	Set 3 TIME	Set 3 REPS
Floor Push-Up Plank						
High Knees in Place						
Floor Oblique Crunch						
Mountain Climbers						

Exercise	Set 4 TIME	Set 4 REPS	Set 5 TIME	Set 5 REPS	Set 6 TIME	Set 6 REPS
Floor Push-Up Plank						
High Knees in Place						
Floor Oblique Crunch						
Mountain Climbers						

Panel 2 — Date: ___ | Routine: Work-to-rest ratio: 60/30 sec.

Exercise	Set 1 TIME	Set 1 REPS	Set 2 TIME	Set 2 REPS	Set 3 TIME	Set 3 REPS
Floor V Crunch (Single Leg)						
Stability Ball Forward Crunch						
Jumping Jacks						
Forward and Backward Jumping						

Exercise	Set 4 TIME	Set 4 REPS	Set 5 TIME	Set 5 REPS	Set 6 TIME	Set 6 REPS
Floor V Crunch (Single Leg)						
Stability Ball Forward Crunch						
Jumping Jacks						
Forward and Backward Jumping						

Panel 3 — Date: ___ | Routine: Work-to-rest ratio: 60/30 sec.

Exercise	Set 1 TIME	Set 1 REPS	Set 2 TIME	Set 2 REPS	Set 3 TIME	Set 3 REPS
Lateral Jumping						
Jump Rope						
Floor Reverse Crunch						
Floor Oblique Crunch						

Exercise	Set 4 TIME	Set 4 REPS	Set 5 TIME	Set 5 REPS	Set 6 TIME	Set 6 REPS
Lateral Jumping						
Jump Rope						
Floor Reverse Crunch						
Floor Oblique Crunch						

Upper and Lower Body

Panel 1 — Date: ___ | Routine: Full Body, Work-to-rest ratio: 60/30 sec.

Exercise	Set 1 LBS	Set 1 REPS	Set 2 LBS	Set 2 REPS	Set 3 LBS	Set 3 REPS
Chin-Ups						
Dumbbell Chest Flies						
Dumbbell Incline Biceps Curl						
Dumbbell Deltoid Frontal Raise						

Exercise	Set 4 LBS	Set 4 REPS	Set 5 LBS	Set 5 REPS	Set 6 LBS	Set 6 REPS
Chin-Ups						
Dumbbell Chest Flies						
Dumbbell Incline Biceps Curl						
Dumbbell Deltoid Frontal Raise						

Panel 2 — Date: ___ | Routine: Lower Body, Work-to-rest ratio: 60/30 sec.

Exercise	Set 1 LBS	Set 1 REPS	Set 2 LBS	Set 2 REPS	Set 3 LBS	Set 3 REPS
Dumbbell Forward Lunges						
Dumbbell Pilates Squat						
Dumbbell Calf Raises						
Dumbbell Squat						

Exercise	Set 4 LBS	Set 4 REPS	Set 5 LBS	Set 5 REPS	Set 6 LBS	Set 6 REPS
Dumbbell Forward Lunges						
Dumbbell Pilates Squat						
Dumbbell Calf Raises						
Dumbbell Squat						

Panel 3 — Date: ___ | Routine: Full Body, Work-to-rest ratio: 60/30 sec.

Exercise	Set 1 LBS	Set 1 REPS	Set 2 LBS	Set 2 REPS	Set 3 LBS	Set 3 REPS
Pull-Ups						
Dumbbell Chest Press						
Dumbbell Sumo Squat						
Dumbbell Back Diagonal Lunges						

Exercise	Set 4 LBS	Set 4 REPS	Set 5 LBS	Set 5 REPS	Set 6 LBS	Set 6 REPS
Pull-Ups						
Dumbbell Chest Press						
Dumbbell Sumo Squat						
Dumbbell Back Diagonal Lunges						

Compound and Functional

Date							Date							Date						
Routine	Work-to-rest ratio: 60/30 sec.						Routine	Work-to-rest ratio: 60/30 sec.						Routine	Work-to-rest ratio: 60/30 sec.					
Exercise	Set 1		Set 2		Set 3		Exercise	Set 1		Set 2		Set 3		Exercise	Set 1		Set 2		Set 3	
	TIME	REPS	TIME	REPS	TIME	REPS		TIME	REPS	TIME	REPS	TIME	REPS		TIME	REPS	TIME	REPS	TIME	REPS
Diagonal Forward Bounding							TRX Suspended Walking Plank							BOSU Reverse Burpee and Roll-Up Squat Hop-Up						
TRX Hack Squat							TRX Suspended Side Plank with Twist							TRX Tornado Twist						
Tuck Jumps							TRX Suspended V Pike							Powerdive Push-Up						
Explosive Start Throws							TRX Suspended Leg Circles							Circle Shoulder Raises						
	Set 4		Set 5		Set 6			Set 4		Set 5		Set 6			Set 4		Set 5		Set 6	
	TIME	REPS	TIME	REPS	TIME	REPS		TIME	REPS	TIME	REPS	TIME	REPS		TIME	REPS	TIME	REPS	TIME	REPS
Diagonal Forward Bounding							TRX Suspended Walking Plank							BOSU Reverse Burpee and Roll-Up Squat Hop-Up						
TRX Hack Squat							TRX Suspended Side Plank with Twist							TRX Tornado Twist						
Tuck Jumps							TRX Suspended V Pike							Powerdive Push-Up						
Explosive Start Throws							TRX Suspended Leg Circles							Circle Shoulder Raises						

Endurance

Mon	Tue	Wed	Thu	Fri	Sat	Sun
Rest or run/ walk	2.75-mile run	Rest or run/ walk	2-mile run	Rest	2.75-mile run	55–60 min. walk

Week 7

You're on the home stretch. With six weeks of training under your belt, you could finish your race now if you had to. These final two weeks will give you that added edge you need to not only *finish* the race but to actually *compete* in it. It's this additional training that will propel you past the weekend warriors and couch potatoes on race day.

Cardio and Core

Date							Date							Date						
Routine	Work-to-rest ratio: 60/15 sec.						Routine	Work-to-rest ratio: 60/15 sec.						Routine	Work-to-rest ratio: 60/15 sec.					
Exercise	Set 1		Set 2		Set 3		Exercise	Set 1		Set 2		Set 3		Exercise	Set 1		Set 2		Set 3	
	TIME	REPS	TIME	REPS	TIME	REPS		TIME	REPS	TIME	REPS	TIME	REPS		TIME	REPS	TIME	REPS	TIME	REPS
Plank Double Leg Lateral Hops							High Knees in Place							Stability Ball Praying Mantis						
Burpees							Burpees							Floor V Crunch (Single Leg)						
Stability Ball Praying Mantis							Forward and Backward Jumping							Floor Pendulum Oblique Twists						
Floor Push-Up Plank							Jump Rope							Floor Reverse Crunch						
	Set 4		Set 5		Set 6			Set 4		Set 5		Set 6			Set 4		Set 5		Set 6	
	TIME	REPS	TIME	REPS	TIME	REPS		TIME	REPS	TIME	REPS	TIME	REPS		TIME	REPS	TIME	REPS	TIME	REPS
Plank Double Leg Lateral Hops							High Knees in Place							Stability Ball Praying Mantis						
Burpees							Burpees							Floor V Crunch (Single Leg)						
Stability Ball Praying Mantis							Forward and Backward Jumping							Floor Pendulum Oblique Twists						
Floor Push-Up Plank							Jump Rope							Floor Reverse Crunch						

Upper and Lower Body

Date							Date							Date						
Routine	Upper Body Time-under-tension: 30 reps in 60 sec.						Routine	Lower Body Time-under-tension: 30 reps in 60 sec.						Routine	Full Body Time-under-tension: 30 reps in 60 sec.					
Exercise	Set 1		Set 2		Set 3		Exercise	Set 1		Set 2		Set 3		Exercise	Set 1		Set 2		Set 3	
	LBS	REPS	LBS	REPS	LBS	REPS		LBS	REPS	LBS	REPS	LBS	REPS		LBS	REPS	LBS	REPS	LBS	REPS
Dumbbell Triceps Kick Back							Dumbbell Sumo Squat							Dumbbell Shoulder Press						
Dumbbell Chest Flies							Dumbbell Calf Raises							Dumbbell Back Rows						
Dumbbell Deltoid Frontal Raise							Butt Hip Raises							Dumbbell Chest Press						
Dumbbell Back Rows							Dumbbell Back Lunges							Dumbbell Squat						
	Set 4		Set 5		Set 6			Set 4		Set 5		Set 6			Set 4		Set 5		Set 6	
	LBS	REPS	LBS	REPS	LBS	REPS		LBS	REPS	LBS	REPS	LBS	REPS		LBS	REPS	LBS	REPS	LBS	REPS
Dumbbell Triceps Kick Back							Dumbbell Sumo Squat							Dumbbell Shoulder Press						
Dumbbell Chest Flies							Dumbbell Calf Raises							Dumbbell Back Rows						
Dumbbell Deltoid Frontal Raise							Butt Hip Raises							Dumbbell Chest Press						
Dumbbell Back Rows							Dumbbell Back Lunges							Dumbbell Squat						

For week seven, continue doing six sets of each exercise with a workout focus as follows: 50 percent power, 30 percent muscular endurance, 20 percent strength. Notice that your work-to-rest ratio really starts putting an emphasis on your increasing endurance, allowing only 15 seconds of rest for every 60 seconds of effort.

Compound and Functional

Date						Date						Date					
Routine	Work-to-rest ratio: 60/15sec.					Routine	Work-to-rest ratio: 60/15sec.					Routine	Work-to-rest ratio: 60/15sec.				
Exercise	Set 1		Set 2		Set 3		Exercise	Set 1		Set 2		Set 3		Exercise	Set 1		Set 2		Set 3
	TIME	REPS	TIME	REPS	TIME	REPS		TIME	REPS	TIME	REPS	TIME	REPS		TIME	REPS	TIME	REPS	TIME	REPS
TRX Atomic Push-Up							TRX Seated Pull-Up							TRX Hack Squat					
Lateral Box Push-Offs							Kneeling to Standing Battling Ropes							TRX Suspended V Pike					
Lateral Hurdle Jumps							BOSU Reverse Burpee and Roll-Up Squat Hop-Up							Explosive Start Throws					
Lateral Jump to Box							TRX Superman							Squat Throws					

(repeated for Set 4, 5, 6)

Endurance

Mon	Tue	Wed	Thu	Fri	Sat	Sun
Rest or run/walk	3-mile run	Rest or run/walk	2-mile run	Rest	3-mile run	60 min. walk

Week 8

Week eight's training focus is 50 percent muscular endurance, 30 percent strength, and 20 percent power. Race day is right around the corner, and because you've been training so diligently you're fully prepared for the challenge. Now go attack those obstacles!

Cardio and Core

Date							Date							Date						
Routine	Work-to-rest ratio: 60/15 sec.						Routine	Work-to-rest ratio: 60/15 sec.						Routine	Work-to-rest ratio: 60/15 sec.					
Exercise	Set 1		Set 2		Set 3		Exercise	Set 1		Set 2		Set 3		Exercise	Set 1		Set 2		Set 3	
	TIME	REPS	TIME	REPS	TIME	REPS		TIME	REPS	TIME	REPS	TIME	REPS		TIME	REPS	TIME	REPS	TIME	REPS
Jump Rope							Burpees							Stability Ball Forward Crunch						
Floor Oblique Crunch							Floor Reverse Crunch							Moutain Climbers						
Mountain Climbers							Power Jacks							Forward and Backward Jumping						
Floor V Crunch (Single Leg)							Floor Oblique Crunch							TRX Side Elbow Plank						
	Set 4		Set 5		Set 6			Set 4		Set 5		Set 6			Set 4		Set 5		Set 6	
	TIME	REPS	TIME	REPS	TIME	REPS		TIME	REPS	TIME	REPS	TIME	REPS		TIME	REPS	TIME	REPS	TIME	REPS
Jump Rope							Burpees							Stability Ball Forward Crunch						
Floor Oblique Crunch							Floor Reverse Crunch							Moutain Climbers						
Mountain Climbers							Power Jacks							Forward and Backward Jumping						
Floor V Crunch (Single Leg)							Floor Oblique Crunch							TRX Side Elbow Plank						

Upper and Lower Body

Date							Date							Date						
Routine	Full Body Work-to-rest ratio: 60/15 sec.						Routine	Lower Body Work-to-rest ratio: 60/15 sec.						Routine	Full Body Work-to-rest ratio: 60/15 sec.					
Exercise	Set 1		Set 2		Set 3		Exercise	Set 1		Set 2		Set 3		Exercise	Set 1		Set 2		Set 3	
	LBS	REPS	LBS	REPS	LBS	REPS		LBS	REPS	LBS	REPS	LBS	REPS		LBS	REPS	LBS	REPS	LBS	REPS
Dumbbell Incline Biceps Curl							Dumbbell Incline Chest Press							Chin-Ups						
Triceps Dips							Side Lying Leg Raises							Dumbbell Sumo Squat						
Pull-Ups							Butt Hip Raises							Dumbbell Back Rows						
Dumbbell Incline Chest Press							Dumbbell Back Lunges							Dumbbell Incline Chest Press						
	Set 4		Set 5		Set 6			Set 4		Set 5		Set 6			Set 4		Set 5		Set 6	
	LBS	REPS	LBS	REPS	LBS	REPS		LBS	REPS	LBS	REPS	LBS	REPS		LBS	REPS	LBS	REPS	LBS	REPS
Dumbbell Incline Biceps Curl							Dumbbell Incline Chest Press							Chin-Ups						
Triceps Dips							Side Lying Leg Raises							Dumbbell Sumo Squat						
Pull-Ups							Butt Hip Raises							Dumbbell Back Rows						
Dumbbell Incline Chest Press							Dumbbell Back Lunges							Dumbbell Incline Chest Press						

Note

You already know that training is going to give you an edge against many other competitors on the obstacle course, but you're going to see the benefits after the race, too: you're not going to have nearly as much postrace fatigue and soreness as folks who did minimal or no training prior to the race.

Compound and Functional

Date							Date							Date						
Routine	Work-to-rest ratio: 60/15 sec.						Routine	Work-to-rest ratio: 60/15 sec.						Routine	Work-to-rest ratio: 60/15 sec.					
Exercise	Set 1		Set 2		Set 3		Exercise	Set 1		Set 2		Set 3		Exercise	Set 1		Set 2		Set 3	
	TIME	REPS	TIME	REPS	TIME	REPS		TIME	REPS	TIME	REPS	TIME	REPS		TIME	REPS	TIME	REPS	TIME	REPS
TRX Suspended Side Plank with Twist and Pike							Lateral Hurdle Jumps							TRX Suspended Side Plank with Twist						
TRX Suspended Walking Plank							Lateral Jump to Box							Tuck Jumps						
BOSU Forward Burpee with Squat Hop-Up Onto BOSU							Circle Shoulder Raises							TRX Atomic Push-Up						
Floor Bear Crawls							BOSU Balance Trainer High Knees with One Leg On and One Leg Off							Diagonal Forward Bounding						
	Set 4		Set 5		Set 6			Set 4		Set 5		Set 6			Set 4		Set 5		Set 6	
	TIME	REPS	TIME	REPS	TIME	REPS		TIME	REPS	TIME	REPS	TIME	REPS		TIME	REPS	TIME	REPS	TIME	REPS
TRX Suspended Side Plank with Twist and Pike							Lateral Hurdle Jumps							TRX Suspended Side Plank with Twist						
TRX Suspended Walking Plank							Lateral Jump to Box							Tuck Jumps						
BOSU Forward Burpee with Squat Hop-Up Onto BOSU							Circle Shoulder Raises							TRX Atomic Push-Up						
Floor Bear Crawls							BOSU Balance Trainer High Knees with One Leg On and One Leg Off							Diagonal Forward Bounding						

Endurance

Mon	Tue	Wed	Thu	Fri	Sat	Sun
Rest or run/walk	3-mile run	Rest or run/walk	2-mile run	Rest	Rest	5k race

Intermediate

If your fitness assessment put you at the intermediate level, you're already in pretty good shape. The eight-week program you are about to embark on is going to start from this solid base and take you to the next level.

Your total training time is 60 minutes (excluding warm-up and endurance training), four days a week. Each day focuses on a different part of your body. Days are broken down as follows:

Day 1—Upper Body:

- Dynamic warm-up (5 minutes)
- Strength training (15 minutes)
- Functional/compound training (15 minutes)
- Cardio training (15 minutes)
- Core training (10 minutes)
- Flexibility (5 minutes)

Day 2—Lower Body:

- Dynamic warm-up (5 minutes)
- Strength training (15 minutes)
- Functional/compound training (15 minutes)
- Cardio training (15 minutes)
- Core training (10 minutes)
- Flexibility (5 minutes)

Day 3—Full Body:

- Dynamic warm-up (5 minutes)
- Strength training (15 minutes)
- Functional/compound training (25 minutes)
- Cardio training (10 minutes)
- Core training (5 minutes)
- Flexibility (5 minutes)

Day 4—Split Training:

- Dynamic warm-up (5 minutes)
- Strength training (15 minutes)
- Functional/compound training (15 minutes)
- Cardio training (15 minutes)
- Core training (10 minutes)
- Flexibility (5 minutes)

Week 1

During week one, perform four sets of each exercise listed on the training worksheets. During your first and second weeks of training, your work-to-rest ratio is dead even: you work for as many seconds as you rest. However, once during each set you're going to do an active rest. An *active rest* is an oxymoron that some demented trainer thought up to mean that you rest the specific muscles that you just worked, but otherwise remain active by doing cardio exercises, such as jumping jacks, jumping rope, or burpees for the duration of your "rest" period. These minicardio sessions are great little tools for taking your endurance and cardiovascular capacity to the next level—without adding time to your total workout. The specific active rest activity is indicated in the Routine section of the training sheet.

The training breakdown for week 1 is as follows: 50 percent neurological adaption, 30 percent strength, 20 percent power.

Cardio and Core

Date						
Routine	Work-to-rest ratio: 45/45 sec.					
Exercise	Set 1		Set 2		Set 3	
	TIME	REPS	TIME	REPS	TIME	REPS
Floor Oblique Crunch						
Jumping Jacks						
Floor Push-Up Plank						
Power Jacks						
	Set 4		Set 5		Set 6	
	TIME	REPS	TIME	REPS	TIME	REPS
Floor Oblique Crunch						
Jumping Jacks						
Floor Push-Up Plank						
Power Jacks						

Date						
Routine	Work-to-rest ratio: 45/45 sec.					
Exercise	Set 1		Set 2		Set 3	
	TIME	REPS	TIME	REPS	TIME	REPS
Floor Pendulum Oblique Twists						
Floor Forward Crunch						
Plank Lateral Jacks						
Jump Rope						
	Set 4		Set 5		Set 6	
	TIME	REPS	TIME	REPS	TIME	REPS
Floor Pendulum Oblique Twists						
Floor Forward Crunch						
Plank Lateral Jacks						
Jump Rope						

Date						
Routine	Work-to-rest ratio: 45/45 sec.					
Exercise	Set 1		Set 2		Set 3	
	TIME	REPS	TIME	REPS	TIME	REPS
Stability Ball Praying Mantis						
Floor V Crunch (Single Leg)						
TRX Side Elbow Plank						
Stability Ball Forward Crunch						
	Set 4		Set 5		Set 6	
	TIME	REPS	TIME	REPS	TIME	REPS
Stability Ball Praying Mantis						
Floor V Crunch (Single Leg)						
TRX Side Elbow Plank						
Stability Ball Forward Crunch						

Date						
Routine	Work-to-rest ratio: 45/45 sec.					
Exercise	Set 1		Set 2		Set 3	
	TIME	REPS	TIME	REPS	TIME	REPS
Jump Rope						
Forward and Backward Jumping						
Lateral Jumping						
High Knees in Place						
	Set 4		Set 5		Set 6	
	TIME	REPS	TIME	REPS	TIME	REPS
Jump Rope						
Forward and Backward Jumping						
Lateral Jumping						
High Knees in Place						

Date						
Routine	Recovery Day					
Exercise	Set 1		Set 2		Set 3	
	TIME	REPS	TIME	REPS	TIME	REPS
	Set 4		Set 5		Set 6	
	TIME	REPS	TIME	REPS	TIME	REPS

Date						
Routine	Recovery Day					
Exercise	Set 1		Set 2		Set 3	
	TIME	REPS	TIME	REPS	TIME	REPS
	Set 4		Set 5		Set 6	
	TIME	REPS	TIME	REPS	TIME	REPS

Upper and Lower Body

Table 1

Date							Date							Date						
Routine	Upper Body — Time-under-tension: 15 reps in 60 sec. Active rest: Jumping Jacks 30 sec. between exercises 2 and 3						Routine	Lower Body — Time-under-tension: 15 reps in 60 sec. Active rest: Jumping Jacks 30 sec. between exercises 1 and 2						Routine	Full Body — Time-under-tension: 15 reps in 60 sec. Active rest: High Knees 30 sec. between exercises 2 and 3					
Exercise	Set 1		Set 2		Set 3		Exercise	Set 1		Set 2		Set 3		Exercise	Set 1		Set 2		Set 3	
	LBS	REPS	LBS	REPS	LBS	REPS		LBS	REPS	LBS	REPS	LBS	REPS		LBS	REPS	LBS	REPS	LBS	REPS
Dumbbell Chest Press							Dumbbell Squat							Dumbbell Incline Chest Press						
Dumbbell Chest Flies							Dumbbell Back Lunges							Dumbbell Sumo Squat						
Dumbbell Back Flies							Side Lying Leg Raises							Dumbbell Shoulder Press						
Dumbbell Back Rows							Butt Hip Raises							Dumbbell Incline Biceps Curl						
	Set 4		Set 5		Set 6			Set 4		Set 5		Set 6			Set 4		Set 5		Set 6	
	LBS	REPS	LBS	REPS	LBS	REPS		LBS	REPS	LBS	REPS	LBS	REPS		LBS	REPS	LBS	REPS	LBS	REPS
Dumbbell Chest Press							Dumbbell Squat							Dumbbell Incline Chest Press						
Dumbbell Chest Flies							Dumbbell Back Lunges							Dumbbell Sumo Squat						
Dumbbell Back Flies							Side Lying Leg Raises							Dumbbell Shoulder Press						
Dumbbell Back Rows							Butt Hip Raises							Dumbbell Incline Biceps Curl						

Table 2

Date							Date							Date						
Routine	Split — Work-to-rest ratio: 45/45 sec. Active rest: Jump Rope 30 sec. between exercises 1 and 2						Routine	Recovery Day						Routine	Recovery Day					
Exercise	Set 1		Set 2		Set 3		Exercise	Set 1		Set 2		Set 3		Exercise	Set 1		Set 2		Set 3	
	LBS	REPS	LBS	REPS	LBS	REPS		LBS	REPS	LBS	REPS	LBS	REPS		LBS	REPS	LBS	REPS	LBS	REPS
Dumbbell Chest Flies																				
Dumbbell Biceps Curl																				
Pull-Ups																				
Chin-Ups																				
	Set 4		Set 5		Set 6			Set 4		Set 5		Set 6			Set 4		Set 5		Set 6	
	LBS	REPS	LBS	REPS	LBS	REPS		LBS	REPS	LBS	REPS	LBS	REPS		LBS	REPS	LBS	REPS	LBS	REPS
Dumbbell Chest Flies																				
Dumbbell Biceps Curl																				
Pull-Ups																				
Chin-Ups																				

Compound and Functional

Block 1

Date						
Routine	Work-to-rest ratio: 60/30 sec. Active rest: Burpees for 30 sec. between exercises 2 and 3					
Exercise	Set 1		Set 2		Set 3	
	TIME	REPS	TIME	REPS	TIME	REPS
TRX Hack Squat						
Lateral Hurdle Jumps						
Powerdive Push-Up						
TRX Seated Pull-Up						
	Set 4		Set 5		Set 6	
	TIME	REPS	TIME	REPS	TIME	REPS
TRX Hack Squat						
Lateral Hurdle Jumps						
Powerdive Push-Up						
TRX Seated Pull-Up						

Block 2

Date						
Routine	Work-to-rest ratio: 60/30 sec. Active rest: Jump Rope for 30 sec. between exercises 2 and 3					
Exercise	Set 1		Set 2		Set 3	
	TIME	REPS	TIME	REPS	TIME	REPS
Forward Hurdle Running						
Sideways Hurdle Running						
Floor Bear Crawls						
Tuck Jumps						
	Set 4		Set 5		Set 6	
	TIME	REPS	TIME	REPS	TIME	REPS
Forward Hurdle Running						
Sideways Hurdle Running						
Floor Bear Crawls						
Tuck Jumps						

Block 3

Date						
Routine	Work-to-rest ratio: 60/30 sec. Active rest: Jumping Jacks for 30 sec. between exercises 1 and 2					
Exercise	Set 1		Set 2		Set 3	
	TIME	REPS	TIME	REPS	TIME	REPS
TRX Suspended Leg Circles						
TRX Suspended V Pike						
TRX Suspended Side Plank with Twist and Pike						
TRX Suspended Side Plank with Twist						
	Set 4		Set 5		Set 6	
	TIME	REPS	TIME	REPS	TIME	REPS
TRX Suspended Leg Circles						
TRX Suspended V Pike						
TRX Suspended Side Plank with Twist and Pike						
TRX Suspended Side Plank with Twist						

Block 4

Date						
Routine	Work-to-rest ratio: 45/45 sec. Active rest: Burpees for 30 sec. between exercises 2 and 3					
Exercise	Set 1		Set 2		Set 3	
	TIME	REPS	TIME	REPS	TIME	REPS
Lateral Hurdle Jumps						
Lateral Jump to Box						
TRX Superman						
Diagonal Forward Bounding						
	Set 4		Set 5		Set 6	
	TIME	REPS	TIME	REPS	TIME	REPS
Lateral Hurdle Jumps						
Lateral Jump to Box						
TRX Superman						
Diagonal Forward Bounding						

Block 5

Date						
Routine	Recovery Day					
Exercise	Set 1		Set 2		Set 3	
	TIME	REPS	TIME	REPS	TIME	REPS
	Set 4		Set 5		Set 6	
	TIME	REPS	TIME	REPS	TIME	REPS

Block 6

Date						
Routine	Recovery Day					
Exercise	Set 1		Set 2		Set 3	
	TIME	REPS	TIME	REPS	TIME	REPS
	Set 4		Set 5		Set 6	
	TIME	REPS	TIME	REPS	TIME	REPS

Endurance

Mon	Tue	Wed	Thu	Fri	Sat	Sun
Rest	3-mile run	5×400	3-mile run	Rest	3-mile run	5-mile run

Week 2

In week two, you continue doing four sets of each exercise. Your training goals for this week's workout are as follows: 50 percent strength, 30 percent power, 20 percent neurological adaptation.

Cardio and Core

Date							Date							Date						
Routine	Work-to-rest ratio: 45/45 sec.						Routine	Work-to-rest ratio: 45/45 sec.						Routine	Work-to-rest ratio: 45/45 sec.					
Exercise	Set 1		Set 2		Set 3		Exercise	Set 1		Set 2		Set 3		Exercise	Set 1		Set 2		Set 3	
	TIME	REPS	TIME	REPS	TIME	REPS		TIME	REPS	TIME	REPS	TIME	REPS		TIME	REPS	TIME	REPS	TIME	REPS
Jumping Jacks							Plank Lateral Jacks							Floor Push-Up Plank						
Stability Ball Praying Mantis							Floor Oblique Crunch							Floor Reverse Crunch						
Burpees							Floor Pendulum Oblique Twists							Mountain Climbers						
Floor Oblique Crunch							Lateral Jumping							Floor Oblique Crunch						

	Set 4		Set 5		Set 6			Set 4		Set 5		Set 6			Set 4		Set 5		Set 6	
	TIME	REPS	TIME	REPS	TIME	REPS		TIME	REPS	TIME	REPS	TIME	REPS		TIME	REPS	TIME	REPS	TIME	REPS
Jumping Jacks							Plank Lateral Jacks							Floor Push-Up Plank						
Stability Ball Praying Mantis							Floor Oblique Crunch							Floor Reverse Crunch						
Burpees							Floor Pendulum Oblique Twists							Mountain Climbers						
Floor Oblique Crunch							Lateral Jumping							Floor Oblique Crunch						

Date							Date							Date						
Routine	Work-to-rest ratio: 45/45 sec.						Routine	Recovery Day						Routine	Recovery Day					
Exercise	Set 1		Set 2		Set 3		Exercise	Set 1		Set 2		Set 3		Exercise	Set 1		Set 2		Set 3	
	TIME	REPS	TIME	REPS	TIME	REPS		TIME	REPS	TIME	REPS	TIME	REPS		TIME	REPS	TIME	REPS	TIME	REPS
Floor Forward Crunch																				
Floor Reverse Crunch																				
Jump Rope																				
Power Jacks																				

	Set 4		Set 5		Set 6			Set 4		Set 5		Set 6			Set 4		Set 5		Set 6	
	TIME	REPS	TIME	REPS	TIME	REPS		TIME	REPS	TIME	REPS	TIME	REPS		TIME	REPS	TIME	REPS	TIME	REPS
Floor Forward Crunch																				
Floor Reverse Crunch																				
Jump Rope																				
Power Jacks																				

Upper and Lower Body

Block 1

Date:

Routine: Upper Body
Work-to-rest ratio: 45/45 sec.
Active rest: Jump Rope 30 sec. between exercises 2 and 3

Exercise	Set 1 LBS	Set 1 REPS	Set 2 LBS	Set 2 REPS	Set 3 LBS	Set 3 REPS
Dumbbell Shoulder Press						
Dumbbell Incline Chest Press						
Triceps Dips						
Chin-Ups						

Exercise	Set 4 LBS	Set 4 REPS	Set 5 LBS	Set 5 REPS	Set 6 LBS	Set 6 REPS
Dumbbell Shoulder Press						
Dumbbell Incline Chest Press						
Triceps Dips						
Chin-Ups						

Block 2

Date:

Routine: Lower Body
Work-to-rest ratio: 45/45 sec.
Active rest: Jumping Jacks 30 sec. between exercises 3 and 4

Exercise	Set 1 LBS	Set 1 REPS	Set 2 LBS	Set 2 REPS	Set 3 LBS	Set 3 REPS
Butt Hip Raises						
Dumbbell Squat						
Dumbbell Calf Raises						
Dumbbell Back Diagonal Lunges						

Exercise	Set 4 LBS	Set 4 REPS	Set 5 LBS	Set 5 REPS	Set 6 LBS	Set 6 REPS
Butt Hip Raises						
Dumbbell Squat						
Dumbbell Calf Raises						
Dumbbell Back Diagonal Lunges						

Block 3

Date:

Routine: Full Body
Work-to-rest ratio: 45/45 sec.
Active rest: High Knees 30 sec. between exercises 2 and 3

Exercise	Set 1 LBS	Set 1 REPS	Set 2 LBS	Set 2 REPS	Set 3 LBS	Set 3 REPS
Dumbbell Chest Press						
Pull-Ups						
Dumbbell Triceps Kick Back						
Dumbbell Back Rows						

Exercise	Set 4 LBS	Set 4 REPS	Set 5 LBS	Set 5 REPS	Set 6 LBS	Set 6 REPS
Dumbbell Chest Press						
Pull-Ups						
Dumbbell Triceps Kick Back						
Dumbbell Back Rows						

Block 4

Date:

Routine: Split
Time-under-tension: 15 reps in 60 sec.
Active rest: Jump Rope 30 sec. between exercises 2 and 3

Exercise	Set 1 LBS	Set 1 REPS	Set 2 LBS	Set 2 REPS	Set 3 LBS	Set 3 REPS
Dumbbell Back Rows						
Dumbbell Back Diagonal Lunges						
Dumbbell Shoulder Press						
Butt Hip Raises						

Exercise	Set 4 LBS	Set 4 REPS	Set 5 LBS	Set 5 REPS	Set 6 LBS	Set 6 REPS
Dumbbell Back Rows						
Dumbbell Back Diagonal Lunges						
Dumbbell Shoulder Press						
Butt Hip Raises						

Block 5

Date:

Routine: Recovery Day

Block 6

Date:

Routine: Recovery Day

Compound and Functional

Date								Date								Date							
Routine	Work-to-rest ratio: 45/45 sec. Active rest: Burpees for 30 sec. between exercises 2 and 3							Routine	Work-to-rest ratio: 45/45 sec. Active rest: Floor Bear Crawls for 30 sec. between exercises 1 and 2							Routine	Work-to-rest ratio: 45/45 sec. Active rest: Jump Rope for 30 sec. between exercises 1 and 2						
Exercise	Set 1		Set 2		Set 3			Exercise	Set 1		Set 2		Set 3			Exercise	Set 1		Set 2		Set 3		
	TIME	REPS	TIME	REPS	TIME	REPS			TIME	REPS	TIME	REPS	TIME	REPS			TIME	REPS	TIME	REPS	TIME	REPS	
TRX Hack Squat								Forward Hurdle Running								TRX Suspended Leg Circles							
Lateral Box Push-Offs								Sideways Hurdle Running								TRX Suspended V Pike							
Powerdive Push-Up								Floor Bear Crawls								TRX Suspended Side Plank with Twist and Pike							
TRX Seated Pull-Up								Tuck Jumps								TRX Suspended Side Plank with Twist							
	Set 4		Set 5		Set 6				Set 4		Set 5		Set 6				Set 4		Set 5		Set 6		
	TIME	REPS	TIME	REPS	TIME	REPS			TIME	REPS	TIME	REPS	TIME	REPS			TIME	REPS	TIME	REPS	TIME	REPS	
TRX Hack Squat								Forward Hurdle Running								TRX Suspended Leg Circles							
Lateral Box Push-Offs								Sideways Hurdle Running								TRX Suspended V Pike							
Powerdive Push-Up								Floor Bear Crawls								TRX Suspended Side Plank with Twist and Pike							
TRX Seated Pull-Up								Tuck Jumps								TRX Suspended Side Plank with Twist							

Date								Date								Date							
Routine	Work-to-rest ratio: 45/45 sec. Active rest: Mountain Climbers for 30 sec. between exercises 2 and 3							Routine	Recovery Day							Routine	Recovery Day						
Exercise	Set 1		Set 2		Set 3			Exercise	Set 1		Set 2		Set 3			Exercise	Set 1		Set 2		Set 3		
	TIME	REPS	TIME	REPS	TIME	REPS			TIME	REPS	TIME	REPS	TIME	REPS			TIME	REPS	TIME	REPS	TIME	REPS	
Lateral Hurdle Jumps																							
Lateral Jump to Box																							
TRX Superman																							
Diagonal Forward Bounding																							
	Set 4		Set 5		Set 6				Set 4		Set 5		Set 6				Set 4		Set 5		Set 6		
	TIME	REPS	TIME	REPS	TIME	REPS			TIME	REPS	TIME	REPS	TIME	REPS			TIME	REPS	TIME	REPS	TIME	REPS	
Lateral Hurdle Jumps																							
Lateral Jump to Box																							
TRX Superman																							
Diagonal Forward Bounding																							

Endurance

Mon	Tue	Wed	Thu	Fri	Sat	Sun
Rest	3-mile run	30 min. tempo	3-mile run	Rest	3-mile fast	5-mile run

Week 3

Week three ups the number of sets to five, and reduces your work-to-rest ratio so that you exercise almost twice as long as you rest. The training goals for this week's workout are 50 percent power, 30 percent muscular endurance, and 20 percent strength.

Cardio and Core

Date							Date							Date						
Routine	Work-to-rest ratio: 50/30 sec.						Routine	Work-to-rest ratio: 50/30 sec.						Routine	Work-to-rest ratio: 50/30 sec.					
Exercise	Set 1		Set 2		Set 3		Exercise	Set 1		Set 2		Set 3		Exercise	Set 1		Set 2		Set 3	
	TIME	REPS	TIME	REPS	TIME	REPS		TIME	REPS	TIME	REPS	TIME	REPS		TIME	REPS	TIME	REPS	TIME	REPS
Floor Push-Up Plank							Forward and Backward Jumping							TRX Side Elbow Plank						
Floor V Crunch (Single Leg)							Power Jacks							High Knees in Place						
Floor Reverse Crunch							Jump Rope							Floor Pendulum Oblique Twists						
Floor Forward Crunch							Lateral Jumping							Forward and Backward Jumping						
	Set 4		Set 5		Set 6			Set 4		Set 5		Set 6			Set 4		Set 5		Set 6	
	TIME	REPS	TIME	REPS	TIME	REPS		TIME	REPS	TIME	REPS	TIME	REPS		TIME	REPS	TIME	REPS	TIME	REPS
Floor Push-Up Plank							Forward and Backward Jumping							TRX Side Elbow Plank						
Floor V Crunch (Single Leg)							Power Jacks							High Knees in Place						
Floor Reverse Crunch							Jump Rope							Floor Pendulum Oblique Twists						
Floor Forward Crunch							Lateral Jumping							Forward and Backward Jumping						

Date							Date							Date						
Routine	Work-to-rest ratio: 50/30 sec.						Routine	Recovery Day						Routine	Recovery Day					
Exercise	Set 1		Set 2		Set 3		Exercise	Set 1		Set 2		Set 3		Exercise	Set 1		Set 2		Set 3	
	TIME	REPS	TIME	REPS	TIME	REPS		TIME	REPS	TIME	REPS	TIME	REPS		TIME	REPS	TIME	REPS	TIME	REPS
Stability Ball Forward Crunch																				
Floor V Crunch (Single Leg)																				
Power Jacks																				
Lateral Jumping																				
	Set 4		Set 5		Set 6			Set 4		Set 5		Set 6			Set 4		Set 5		Set 6	
	TIME	REPS	TIME	REPS	TIME	REPS		TIME	REPS	TIME	REPS	TIME	REPS		TIME	REPS	TIME	REPS	TIME	REPS
Stability Ball Forward Crunch																				
Floor V Crunch (Single Leg)																				
Power Jacks																				
Lateral Jumping																				

Upper and Lower Body

Table 1 (Upper Body)

Date	
Routine	Upper Body. Time-under-tension: 15 reps in 60 sec. Active rest: Jump Rope 30 sec. between exercises 1 and 2

Exercise	Set 1 LBS	Set 1 REPS	Set 2 LBS	Set 2 REPS	Set 3 LBS	Set 3 REPS
Dumbbell Triceps Kick Back						
Dumbbell Incline Chest Press						
Dumbbell Shoulder Press						
Chin-Ups						

	Set 4 LBS	Set 4 REPS	Set 5 LBS	Set 5 REPS	Set 6 LBS	Set 6 REPS
Dumbbell Triceps Kick Back						
Dumbbell Incline Chest Press						
Dumbbell Shoulder Press						
Chin-Ups						

Table 2 (Lower Body)

Date	
Routine	Lower Body. Time-under-tension: 15 reps in 60 sec. Active rest: Jumping Jacks 30 sec. between exercises 1 and 2

Exercise	Set 1 LBS	Set 1 REPS	Set 2 LBS	Set 2 REPS	Set 3 LBS	Set 3 REPS
Dumbbell Pilates Squat						
Side Lying Leg Raises						
Dumbbell Back Lunges						
Butt Hip Raises						

	Set 4 LBS	Set 4 REPS	Set 5 LBS	Set 5 REPS	Set 6 LBS	Set 6 REPS
Dumbbell Pilates Squat						
Side Lying Leg Raises						
Dumbbell Back Lunges						
Butt Hip Raises						

Table 3 (Full Body)

Date	
Routine	Full Body. Time-under-tension: 15 reps in 60 sec. Active rest: High Knees 30 sec. between exercises 3 and 4

Exercise	Set 1 LBS	Set 1 REPS	Set 2 LBS	Set 2 REPS	Set 3 LBS	Set 3 REPS
Dumbbell Chest Flies						
Dumbbell Squat						
Dumbbell Back Flies						
Dumbbell Back Diagonal Lunges						

	Set 4 LBS	Set 4 REPS	Set 5 LBS	Set 5 REPS	Set 6 LBS	Set 6 REPS
Dumbbell Chest Flies						
Dumbbell Squat						
Dumbbell Back Flies						
Dumbbell Back Diagonal Lunges						

Table 4 (Split)

Date	
Routine	Split. Work-to-rest ratio: 50/30 sec. Active rest: Jump Rope 30 sec. between exercises 2 and 3

Exercise	Set 1 LBS	Set 1 REPS	Set 2 LBS	Set 2 REPS	Set 3 LBS	Set 3 REPS
Dumbbell Chest Flies						
Dumbbell Back Flies						
Side Lying Leg Raises						
Butt Hip Raises						

	Set 4 LBS	Set 4 REPS	Set 5 LBS	Set 5 REPS	Set 6 LBS	Set 6 REPS
Dumbbell Chest Flies						
Dumbbell Back Flies						
Side Lying Leg Raises						
Butt Hip Raises						

Table 5 (Recovery Day)

Date	
Routine	Recovery Day

Exercise	Set 1 LBS	Set 1 REPS	Set 2 LBS	Set 2 REPS	Set 3 LBS	Set 3 REPS

	Set 4 LBS	Set 4 REPS	Set 5 LBS	Set 5 REPS	Set 6 LBS	Set 6 REPS

Table 6 (Recovery Day)

Date	
Routine	Recovery Day

Exercise	Set 1 LBS	Set 1 REPS	Set 2 LBS	Set 2 REPS	Set 3 LBS	Set 3 REPS

	Set 4 LBS	Set 4 REPS	Set 5 LBS	Set 5 REPS	Set 6 LBS	Set 6 REPS

Compound and Functional

Date							Date							Date						
Routine	Work-to-rest ratio: 50/30 sec. Active rest: Burpees for 30 sec. between exercises 2 and 3						Routine	Work-to-rest ratio: 50/30 sec. Active rest: Floor Bear Crawls for 30 sec. between exercises 1 and 2						Routine	Work-to-rest ratio: 50/30 sec. Active rest: Jump Rope for 30 sec. between exercises 1 and 2					
Exercise	Set 1		Set 2		Set 3		Exercise	Set 1		Set 2		Set 3		Exercise	Set 1		Set 2		Set 3	
	TIME	REPS	TIME	REPS	TIME	REPS		TIME	REPS	TIME	REPS	TIME	REPS		TIME	REPS	TIME	REPS	TIME	REPS
TRX Atomic Push-Up							Explosive Start Throws							BOSU Balance Trainer High Knees with One Leg On and One Leg Off						
TRX Suspended V Pike							BOSU Reverse Burpee and Roll-Up Squat Hop-Up							TRX Suspended Side Plank with Twist and Pike						
TRX Atomic Push-Up							TRX Hack Squat							Sideways Hurdle Running						
TRX Tornado Twist							TRX Suspended Side Plank with Twist							Powerdive Push-Up						
	Set 4		Set 5		Set 6			Set 4		Set 5		Set 6			Set 4		Set 5		Set 6	
	TIME	REPS	TIME	REPS	TIME	REPS		TIME	REPS	TIME	REPS	TIME	REPS		TIME	REPS	TIME	REPS	TIME	REPS
TRX Atomic Push-Up							Explosive Start Throws							BOSU Balance Trainer High Knees with One Leg On and One Leg Off						
TRX Suspended V Pike							BOSU Reverse Burpee and Roll-Up Squat Hop-Up							TRX Suspended Side Plank with Twist and Pike						
TRX Atomic Push-Up							TRX Hack Squat							Sideways Hurdle Running						
TRX Tornado Twist							TRX Suspended Side Plank with Twist							Powerdive Push-Up						

Date							Date							Date						
Routine	Work-to-rest ratio: 50/30 sec. Active rest: Burpees for 30 sec. between exercises 2 and 3						Routine	Recovery Day						Routine	Recovery Day					
Exercise	Set 1		Set 2		Set 3		Exercise	Set 1		Set 2		Set 3		Exercise	Set 1		Set 2		Set 3	
	TIME	REPS	TIME	REPS	TIME	REPS		TIME	REPS	TIME	REPS	TIME	REPS		TIME	REPS	TIME	REPS	TIME	REPS
Forward Hurdle Running																				
Floor Bear Crawls																				
Diagonal Forward Bounding																				
Powerdive Push-Up																				
	Set 4		Set 5		Set 6			Set 4		Set 5		Set 6			Set 4		Set 5		Set 6	
	TIME	REPS	TIME	REPS	TIME	REPS		TIME	REPS	TIME	REPS	TIME	REPS		TIME	REPS	TIME	REPS	TIME	REPS
Forward Hurdle Running																				
Floor Bear Crawls																				
Diagonal Forward Bounding																				
Powerdive Push-Up																				

Endurance

Mon	Tue	Wed	Thu	Fri	Sat	Sun
Rest	3-mile run	6×400	3-mile run	Rest	4-mile run	6-mile run

Week 4

By week four, you should feel completely energized by your workouts. You're getting stronger by the day, and are gaining the endurance and cardiovascular fitness you need to wage an all-out attack on the racing portion of the obstacle course. If you're combining your workout with a low-calorie, nutritious diet, you might even be shedding some weight.

The workouts for this week focus on 50 percent strength, 30 percent muscular endurance, and 20 percent power.

Cardio and Core

Date							Date							Date						
Routine	Work-to-rest ratio: 50/30 sec.						Routine	Work-to-rest ratio: 50/30 sec.						Routine	Work-to-rest ratio: 50/30 sec.					
Exercise	Set 1		Set 2		Set 3		Exercise	Set 1		Set 2		Set 3		Exercise	Set 1		Set 2		Set 3	
	TIME	REPS	TIME	REPS	TIME	REPS		TIME	REPS	TIME	REPS	TIME	REPS		TIME	REPS	TIME	REPS	TIME	REPS
Stability Ball Praying Mantis							Floor Oblique Crunch							Floor Forward Crunch						
Jump Rope							Burpees							High Knees in Place						
Floor Reverse Crunch							Floor Push-Up Plank							Mountain Climbers						
Forward and Backward Jumping							Lateral Jumping							Floor V Crunch (Single Leg)						
	Set 4		Set 5		Set 6			Set 4		Set 5		Set 6			Set 4		Set 5		Set 6	
	TIME	REPS	TIME	REPS	TIME	REPS		TIME	REPS	TIME	REPS	TIME	REPS		TIME	REPS	TIME	REPS	TIME	REPS
Stability Ball Praying Mantis							Floor Oblique Crunch							Floor Forward Crunch						
Jump Rope							Burpees							High Knees in Place						
Floor Reverse Crunch							Floor Push-Up Plank							Mountain Climbers						
Forward and Backward Jumping							Lateral Jumping							Floor V Crunch (Single Leg)						

Date							Date							Date						
Routine	Work-to-rest ratio: 50/30 sec.						Routine	Recovery Day						Routine	Recovery Day					
Exercise	Set 1		Set 2		Set 3		Exercise	Set 1		Set 2		Set 3		Exercise	Set 1		Set 2		Set 3	
	TIME	REPS	TIME	REPS	TIME	REPS		TIME	REPS	TIME	REPS	TIME	REPS		TIME	REPS	TIME	REPS	TIME	REPS
Plank Double Leg Lateral Hops																				
Floor Pendulum Oblique Twists																				
Jump Rope																				
Floor Push-Up Plank																				
	Set 4		Set 5		Set 6			Set 4		Set 5		Set 6			Set 4		Set 5		Set 6	
	TIME	REPS	TIME	REPS	TIME	REPS		TIME	REPS	TIME	REPS	TIME	REPS		TIME	REPS	TIME	REPS	TIME	REPS
Plank Double Leg Lateral Hops																				
Floor Pendulum Oblique Twists																				
Jump Rope																				
Floor Push-Up Plank																				

Upper and Lower Body

Date			Date			Date		
Routine	Upper Body. Work-to-rest ratio: 50/30 sec. Active rest: Jump Rope 30 sec. between exercises 1 and 2		**Routine**	Lower Body. Work-to-rest ratio: 50/30 sec. Active rest: Jumping Jacks 30 sec. between exercises 2 and 3		**Routine**	Full Body. Work-to-rest ratio: 50/30 sec. Active rest: High Knees 30 sec. between exercises 2 and 3	

Exercise	Set 1 (LBS/REPS)	Set 2 (LBS/REPS)	Set 3 (LBS/REPS)	Exercise	Set 1 (LBS/REPS)	Set 2 (LBS/REPS)	Set 3 (LBS/REPS)	Exercise	Set 1 (LBS/REPS)	Set 2 (LBS/REPS)	Set 3 (LBS/REPS)
Dumbbell Chest Press				Dumbbell Sumo Squat				Dumbbell Biceps Curl			
Triceps Dips				Dumbbell Back Lunges				Triceps Dips			
Dumbbell Deltoid Lateral Raise				Dumbbell Calf Raises				Dumbbell Squat			
Dumbbell Deltoid Frontal Raise				Side Lying Leg Raises				Dumbbell Back Lunges			

Exercise	Set 4 (LBS/REPS)	Set 5 (LBS/REPS)	Set 6 (LBS/REPS)	Exercise	Set 4 (LBS/REPS)	Set 5 (LBS/REPS)	Set 6 (LBS/REPS)	Exercise	Set 4 (LBS/REPS)	Set 5 (LBS/REPS)	Set 6 (LBS/REPS)
Dumbbell Chest Press				Dumbbell Sumo Squat				Dumbbell Biceps Curl			
Triceps Dips				Dumbbell Back Lunges				Triceps Dips			
Dumbbell Deltoid Lateral Raise				Dumbbell Calf Raises				Dumbbell Squat			
Dumbbell Deltoid Frontal Raise				Side Lying Leg Raises				Dumbbell Back Lunges			

Date			Date			Date		
Routine	Split. Time-under-tension: 15 reps in 60 sec. Active rest: Jump Rope 30 sec. between exercises 1 and 2		**Routine**	Recovery Day		**Routine**	Recovery Day	

Exercise	Set 1 (LBS/REPS)	Set 2 (LBS/REPS)	Set 3 (LBS/REPS)	Exercise	Set 1 (LBS/REPS)	Set 2 (LBS/REPS)	Set 3 (LBS/REPS)	Exercise	Set 1 (LBS/REPS)	Set 2 (LBS/REPS)	Set 3 (LBS/REPS)
Dumbbell Biceps Curl											
Triceps Dips											
Dumbbell Squat											
Dumbbell Back Lunges											

Exercise	Set 4 (LBS/REPS)	Set 5 (LBS/REPS)	Set 6 (LBS/REPS)	Exercise	Set 4 (LBS/REPS)	Set 5 (LBS/REPS)	Set 6 (LBS/REPS)	Exercise	Set 4 (LBS/REPS)	Set 5 (LBS/REPS)	Set 6 (LBS/REPS)
Dumbbell Biceps Curl											
Triceps Dips											
Dumbbell Squat											
Dumbbell Back Lunges											

Tip

Now that you've been training for four full weeks, take the Fitness Level Assessment located earlier in this chapter to check on your progress and see if you should bump up (or down) to the next fitness level.

Compound and Functional

Date							Date							Date						
Routine	Work-to-rest ratio: 55/20 sec. Active rest: Burpees for 30 sec. between exercises 2 and 3						Routine	Work-to-rest ratio: 55/20 sec. Active rest: Jump Rope for 30 sec. between exercises 2 and 3						Routine	Work-to-rest ratio: 55/20 sec. Active rest: Jumping Jacks for 30 sec. between exercises 1 and 2					
Exercise	Set 1		Set 2		Set 3		Exercise	Set 1		Set 2		Set 3		Exercise	Set 1		Set 2		Set 3	
	TIME	REPS	TIME	REPS	TIME	REPS		TIME	REPS	TIME	REPS	TIME	REPS		TIME	REPS	TIME	REPS	TIME	REPS
Lateral Jump to Box							TRX Suspended V Pike							TRX Suspended Leg Circles						
Squat Throws							TRX Hack Squat							TRX Suspended Walking Plank						
Circle Shoulder Raises							Floor Bear Crawls							TRX Atomic Push-Up						
Tuck Jumps							Kneeling to Standing Battling Ropes							TRX Superman						
	Set 4		Set 5		Set 6			Set 4		Set 5		Set 6			Set 4		Set 5		Set 6	
	TIME	REPS	TIME	REPS	TIME	REPS		TIME	REPS	TIME	REPS	TIME	REPS		TIME	REPS	TIME	REPS	TIME	REPS
Lateral Jump to Box							TRX Suspended V Pike							TRX Suspended Leg Circles						
Squat Throws							TRX Hack Squat							TRX Suspended Walking Plank						
Circle Shoulder Raises							Floor Bear Crawls							TRX Atomic Push-Up						
Tuck Jumps							Kneeling to Standing Battling Ropes							TRX Superman						

Date							Date							Date						
Routine	Work-to-rest ratio: 50/30 sec. Active rest: Mountain Climbers for 30 sec. between exercises 2 and 3						Routine	Recovery Day						Routine	Recovery Day					
Exercise	Set 1		Set 2		Set 3		Exercise	Set 1		Set 2		Set 3		Exercise	Set 1		Set 2		Set 3	
	TIME	REPS	TIME	REPS	TIME	REPS		TIME	REPS	TIME	REPS	TIME	REPS		TIME	REPS	TIME	REPS	TIME	REPS
TRX Superman																				
TRX Atomic Push-Up																				
Tuck Jumps																				
BOSU Forward Burpee with Squat Hop-Up Onto BOSU																				
	Set 4		Set 5		Set 6			Set 4		Set 5		Set 6			Set 4		Set 5		Set 6	
	TIME	REPS	TIME	REPS	TIME	REPS		TIME	REPS	TIME	REPS	TIME	REPS		TIME	REPS	TIME	REPS	TIME	REPS
TRX Superman																				
TRX Atomic Push-Up																				
Tuck Jumps																				
BOSU Forward Burpee with Squat Hop-Up Onto BOSU																				

Endurance

Mon	Tue	Wed	Thu	Fri	Sat	Sun
Rest	3-mile run	35 min. tempo	3-mile run	Rest	Rest	5k test

Week 5

In week five you pull out all the stops, with six full sets of each exercise and very little rest between each. Soon you will be an obstacle-racing machine.

Cardio and Core

Block 1

Date						
Routine	Work-to-rest ratio: 55/20 sec.					
Exercise	Set 1		Set 2		Set 3	
	TIME	REPS	TIME	REPS	TIME	REPS
Mountain Climbers						
Floor V Crunch (Single Leg)						
Floor Reverse Crunch						
Power Jacks						
	Set 4		Set 5		Set 6	
	TIME	REPS	TIME	REPS	TIME	REPS
Mountain Climbers						
Floor V Crunch (Single Leg)						
Floor Reverse Crunch						
Power Jacks						

Block 2

Date						
Routine	Work-to-rest ratio: 55/20 sec.					
Exercise	Set 1		Set 2		Set 3	
	TIME	REPS	TIME	REPS	TIME	REPS
Jumping Jacks						
Burpees						
Floor Oblique Crunch						
Floor Pendulum Oblique Twists						
	Set 4		Set 5		Set 6	
	TIME	REPS	TIME	REPS	TIME	REPS
Jumping Jacks						
Burpees						
Floor Oblique Crunch						
Floor Pendulum Oblique Twists						

Block 3

Date						
Routine	Work-to-rest ratio: 55/20 sec.					
Exercise	Set 1		Set 2		Set 3	
	TIME	REPS	TIME	REPS	TIME	REPS
Lateral Jumping						
Floor Forward Crunch						
Stability Ball Forward Crunch						
Plank Lateral Jacks						
	Set 4		Set 5		Set 6	
	TIME	REPS	TIME	REPS	TIME	REPS
Lateral Jumping						
Floor Forward Crunch						
Stability Ball Forward Crunch						
Plank Lateral Jacks						

Block 4

Date						
Routine	Work-to-rest ratio: 55/20 sec.					
Exercise	Set 1		Set 2		Set 3	
	TIME	REPS	TIME	REPS	TIME	REPS
High Knees in Place						
Burpees						
Floor V Crunch (Single Leg)						
Floor Push-Up Plank						
	Set 4		Set 5		Set 6	
	TIME	REPS	TIME	REPS	TIME	REPS
High Knees in Place						
Burpees						
Floor V Crunch (Single Leg)						
Floor Push-Up Plank						

Block 5

Date						
Routine	Recovery Day					
Exercise	Set 1		Set 2		Set 3	
	TIME	REPS	TIME	REPS	TIME	REPS
	Set 4		Set 5		Set 6	
	TIME	REPS	TIME	REPS	TIME	REPS

Block 6

Date						
Routine	Recovery Day					
Exercise	Set 1		Set 2		Set 3	
	TIME	REPS	TIME	REPS	TIME	REPS
	Set 4		Set 5		Set 6	
	TIME	REPS	TIME	REPS	TIME	REPS

Upper and Lower Body

Date						
Routine	Upper Body Time-under-tension: 20 reps in 60 sec. Active rest: Mountain Climbers 30 sec. between exercises 1 and 2					

Exercise	Set 1		Set 2		Set 3	
	LBS	REPS	LBS	REPS	LBS	REPS
Dumbbell Incline Chest Press						
Chin-Ups						
Dumbbell Shoulder Press						
Dumbbell Triceps Skull Crusher						

	Set 4		Set 5		Set 6	
	LBS	REPS	LBS	REPS	LBS	REPS
Dumbbell Incline Chest Press						
Chin-Ups						
Dumbbell Shoulder Press						
Dumbbell Triceps Skull Crusher						

Date						
Routine	Lower Body Time-under-tension: 20 reps in 60 sec. Active rest: High Knees 30 sec. between exercises 1 and 2					

Exercise	Set 1		Set 2		Set 3	
	LBS	REPS	LBS	REPS	LBS	REPS
Dumbbell Calf Raises						
Dumbbell Squat						
Dumbbell Forward Lunges						
Dumbbell Pilates Squat						

	Set 4		Set 5		Set 6	
	LBS	REPS	LBS	REPS	LBS	REPS
Dumbbell Calf Raises						
Dumbbell Squat						
Dumbbell Forward Lunges						
Dumbbell Pilates Squat						

Date						
Routine	Full Body Time-under-tension: 20 reps in 60 sec. Active rest: Burpees 30 sec. between exercises 3 and 4					

Exercise	Set 1		Set 2		Set 3	
	LBS	REPS	LBS	REPS	LBS	REPS
Dumbbell Triceps Overhead Extension						
Dumbbell Incline Biceps Curl						
Dumbbell Squat						
Dumbbell Back Lunges						

	Set 4		Set 5		Set 6	
	LBS	REPS	LBS	REPS	LBS	REPS
Dumbbell Triceps Overhead Extension						
Dumbbell Incline Biceps Curl						
Dumbbell Squat						
Dumbbell Back Lunges						

Date						
Routine	Split Work-to-rest ratio: 60/20 sec. Active rest: Jump Rope 30 sec. between exercises 2 and 3					

Exercise	Set 1		Set 2		Set 3	
	LBS	REPS	LBS	REPS	LBS	REPS
Dumbbell Pilates Squat						
Pull-Ups						
Butt Hip Raises						
Dumbbell Back Rows						

	Set 4		Set 5		Set 6	
	LBS	REPS	LBS	REPS	LBS	REPS
Dumbbell Pilates Squat						
Pull-Ups						
Butt Hip Raises						
Dumbbell Back Rows						

Date						
Routine	Recovery Day					

Exercise	Set 1		Set 2		Set 3	
	LBS	REPS	LBS	REPS	LBS	REPS

	Set 4		Set 5		Set 6	
	LBS	REPS	LBS	REPS	LBS	REPS

Date						
Routine	Recovery Day					

Exercise	Set 1		Set 2		Set 3	
	LBS	REPS	LBS	REPS	LBS	REPS

	Set 4		Set 5		Set 6	
	LBS	REPS	LBS	REPS	LBS	REPS

Compound and Functional

Routine 1

Date						
Routine	Work-to-rest ratio: 55/20 sec. Active rest: Burpees for 30 sec. between exercises 2 and 3					

Exercise	Set 1 TIME	Set 1 REPS	Set 2 TIME	Set 2 REPS	Set 3 TIME	Set 3 REPS
Lateral Jump to Box						
Squat Throws						
Circle Shoulder Raises						
Tuck Jumps						

Exercise	Set 4 TIME	Set 4 REPS	Set 5 TIME	Set 5 REPS	Set 6 TIME	Set 6 REPS
Lateral Jump to Box						
Squat Throws						
Circle Shoulder Raises						
Tuck Jumps						

Routine 2

Date						
Routine	Work-to-rest ratio: 55/20 sec. Active rest: Jump Rope for 30 sec. between exercises 2 and 3					

Exercise	Set 1 TIME	Set 1 REPS	Set 2 TIME	Set 2 REPS	Set 3 TIME	Set 3 REPS
TRX Suspended V Pike						
TRX Hack Squat						
Floor Bear Crawls						
Kneeling to Standing Battling Ropes						

Exercise	Set 4 TIME	Set 4 REPS	Set 5 TIME	Set 5 REPS	Set 6 TIME	Set 6 REPS
TRX Suspended V Pike						
TRX Hack Squat						
Floor Bear Crawls						
Kneeling to Standing Battling Ropes						

Routine 3

Date						
Routine	Work-to-rest ratio: 55/20 sec. Active rest: Jumping Jacks for 30 sec. between exercises 1 and 2					

Exercise	Set 1 TIME	Set 1 REPS	Set 2 TIME	Set 2 REPS	Set 3 TIME	Set 3 REPS
TRX Suspended Leg Circles						
TRX Suspended Walking Plank						
TRX Atomic Push-Up						
TRX Superman						

Exercise	Set 4 TIME	Set 4 REPS	Set 5 TIME	Set 5 REPS	Set 6 TIME	Set 6 REPS
TRX Suspended Leg Circles						
TRX Suspended Walking Plank						
TRX Atomic Push-Up						
TRX Superman						

Routine 4

Date						
Routine	Work-to-rest ratio: 55/20 sec. Active rest: Burpees for 30 sec. between exercises 2 and 3					

Exercise	Set 1 TIME	Set 1 REPS	Set 2 TIME	Set 2 REPS	Set 3 TIME	Set 3 REPS
Lateral Hurdle Jumps						
BOSU Forward Burpee with Squat Hop-Up Onto BOSU						
Powerdive Push-Up						
Pull-Ups						

Exercise	Set 4 TIME	Set 4 REPS	Set 5 TIME	Set 5 REPS	Set 6 TIME	Set 6 REPS
Lateral Hurdle Jumps						
BOSU Forward Burpee with Squat Hop-Up Onto BOSU						
Powerdive Push-Up						
Pull-Ups						

Recovery Day

Date		Routine: Recovery Day

Recovery Day

Date		Routine: Recovery Day

Endurance

Mon	Tue	Wed	Thu	Fri	Sat	Sun
Rest	3-mile run	7×400	3-mile run	Rest	4-mile fast	6-mile run

Week 6

Continue attacking your sets and maximizing your endurance training in week six. Your fitness goals for this week are as follows: 50 percent strength, 30 percent power, 20 percent muscular endurance.

Cardio and Core

Date							Date							Date						
Routine	Work-to-rest ratio: 55/20 sec.						Routine	Work-to-rest ratio: 55/20 sec.						Routine	Work-to-rest ratio: 55/20 sec.					
Exercise	Set 1		Set 2		Set 3		Exercise	Set 1		Set 2		Set 3		Exercise	Set 1		Set 2		Set 3	
	TIME	REPS	TIME	REPS	TIME	REPS		TIME	REPS	TIME	REPS	TIME	REPS		TIME	REPS	TIME	REPS	TIME	REPS
Floor Oblique Crunch							Jumping Jacks							Floor Forward Crunch						
TRX Side Elbow Plank							High Knees in Place							Plank Double Leg Lateral Hops						
Floor V Crunch (Single Leg)							Floor Reverse Crunch							Floor Pendulum Oblique Twists						
Burpees							Forward and Backward Jumping							Floor Oblique Crunch						
	Set 4		Set 5		Set 6			Set 4		Set 5		Set 6			Set 4		Set 5		Set 6	
	TIME	REPS	TIME	REPS	TIME	REPS		TIME	REPS	TIME	REPS	TIME	REPS		TIME	REPS	TIME	REPS	TIME	REPS
Floor Oblique Crunch							Jumping Jacks							Floor Forward Crunch						
TRX Side Elbow Plank							High Knees in Place							Plank Double Leg Lateral Hops						
Floor V Crunch (Single Leg)							Floor Reverse Crunch							Floor Pendulum Oblique Twists						
Burpees							Forward and Backward Jumping							Floor Oblique Crunch						

Date							Date							Date						
Routine	Work-to-rest ratio: 55/20 sec.						Routine	Recovery Day						Routine	Recovery Day					
Exercise	Set 1		Set 2		Set 3		Exercise	Set 1		Set 2		Set 3		Exercise	Set 1		Set 2		Set 3	
	TIME	REPS	TIME	REPS	TIME	REPS		TIME	REPS	TIME	REPS	TIME	REPS		TIME	REPS	TIME	REPS	TIME	REPS
Burpees																				
Jump Rope																				
Stability Ball Forward Crunch																				
Floor Oblique Crunch																				
	Set 4		Set 5		Set 6			Set 4		Set 5		Set 6			Set 4		Set 5		Set 6	
	TIME	REPS	TIME	REPS	TIME	REPS		TIME	REPS	TIME	REPS	TIME	REPS		TIME	REPS	TIME	REPS	TIME	REPS
Burpees																				
Jump Rope																				
Stability Ball Forward Crunch																				
Floor Oblique Crunch																				

Upper and Lower Body

Date						Date						Date					
Routine	Upper Body Work-to-rest ratio: 60/20 sec. Active rest: Jump Rope 30 sec. between exercises 1 and 2					Routine	Lower Body Work-to-rest ratio: 60/20 sec. Active rest: Jumping Jacks 30 sec. between exercises 2 and 3					Routine	Full Body Work-to-rest ratio: 60/20 sec. Active rest: High Knees 30 sec. between exercises 2 and 3				
Exercise	Set 1		Set 2		Set 3	Exercise	Set 1		Set 2		Set 3	Exercise	Set 1		Set 2		Set 3
	LBS	REPS	LBS	REPS	LBS	REPS		LBS	REPS	LBS	REPS	LBS	REPS		LBS	REPS	LBS	REPS

(Set 1 / Set 2 / Set 3 columns, each with LBS and REPS)

First block — Sets 1–3

Exercise (Upper)	Exercise (Lower)	Exercise (Full)
Triceps Dips	Dumbbell Sumo Squat	Dumbbell Incline Chest Press
Dumbbell Biceps Curl	Side Lying Leg Raises	Dumbbell Back Flies
Chin-Ups	Dumbbell Calf Raises	Dumbbell Squat
Dumbbell Shoulder Press	Dumbbell Back Diagonal Lunges	Side Lying Leg Raises

First block — Sets 4–6

Exercise (Upper)	Exercise (Lower)	Exercise (Full)
Triceps Dips	Dumbbell Sumo Squat	Dumbbell Incline Chest Press
Dumbbell Biceps Curl	Side Lying Leg Raises	Dumbbell Back Flies
Chin-Ups	Dumbbell Calf Raises	Dumbbell Squat
Dumbbell Shoulder Press	Dumbbell Back Diagonal Lunges	Side Lying Leg Raises

Second block

Routine	Split Time-under-tension: 20 reps in 60 sec. Active rest: Jumping Jacks 30 sec. between exercises 1 and 2	Routine	Recovery Day	Routine	Recovery Day

Sets 1–3 and Sets 4–6

Exercise (Split)
Dumbbell Deltoid Lateral Raise
Dumbbell Forward Lunges
Dumbbell Triceps Kick Back
Dumbbell Pilates Squat

Endurance

Mon	Tue	Wed	Thu	Fri	Sat	Sun
Rest	3-mile run	40 min. tempo	3-mile run	Rest	5-mile run	7-mile run

Compound and Functional

Routine 1

Date:

Routine: Work-to-rest ratio: 55/20 sec. Active rest: Burpees for 30 sec. between exercises 2 and 3

Exercise	Set 1		Set 2		Set 3	
	TIME	REPS	TIME	REPS	TIME	REPS
Diagonal Forward Bounding						
TRX Hack Squat						
TRX Atomic Push-Up						
Sideways Hurdle Running						

Exercise	Set 4		Set 5		Set 6	
	TIME	REPS	TIME	REPS	TIME	REPS
Diagonal Forward Bounding						
TRX Hack Squat						
TRX Atomic Push-Up						
Sideways Hurdle Running						

Routine 2

Date:

Routine: Work-to-rest ratio: 55/20 sec. Active rest: Floor Bear Crawls for 30 sec. between exercises 1 and 2

Exercise	Set 1		Set 2		Set 3	
	TIME	REPS	TIME	REPS	TIME	REPS
TRX Suspended Side Plank with Twist						
TRX Atomic Push-Up						
TRX Superman						
TRX Suspended Walking Plank						

Exercise	Set 4		Set 5		Set 6	
	TIME	REPS	TIME	REPS	TIME	REPS
TRX Suspended Side Plank with Twist						
TRX Atomic Push-Up						
TRX Superman						
TRX Suspended Walking Plank						

Routine 3

Date:

Routine: Work-to-rest ratio: 55/20 sec. Active rest: Jump Rope for 30 sec. between exercises 1 and 2

Exercise	Set 1		Set 2		Set 3	
	TIME	REPS	TIME	REPS	TIME	REPS
TRX Suspended V Pike						
TRX Suspended Side Plank with Twist and Pike						
BOSU Reverse Burpee and Roll-Up Squat Hop-Up						
BOSU Balance Trainer High Knees with One Leg On and One Leg Off						

Exercise	Set 4		Set 5		Set 6	
	TIME	REPS	TIME	REPS	TIME	REPS
TRX Suspended V Pike						
TRX Suspended Side Plank with Twist and Pike						
BOSU Reverse Burpee and Roll-Up Squat Hop-Up						
BOSU Balance Trainer High Knees with One Leg On and One Leg Off						

Routine 4

Date:

Routine: Work-to-rest ratio: 55/20 sec. Active rest: Mountain Climbers for 30 sec. between exercises 2 and 3

Exercise	Set 1		Set 2		Set 3	
	TIME	REPS	TIME	REPS	TIME	REPS
Lateral Jump to Box						
Forward Hurdle Running						
Circle Shoulder Raises						
Powerdive Push-Up						

Exercise	Set 4		Set 5		Set 6	
	TIME	REPS	TIME	REPS	TIME	REPS
Lateral Jump to Box						
Forward Hurdle Running						
Circle Shoulder Raises						
Powerdive Push-Up						

Routine 5

Date:

Routine: Recovery Day

Exercise	Set 1		Set 2		Set 3	
	TIME	REPS	TIME	REPS	TIME	REPS

Exercise	Set 4		Set 5		Set 6	
	TIME	REPS	TIME	REPS	TIME	REPS

Routine 6

Date:

Routine: Recovery Day

Exercise	Set 1		Set 2		Set 3	
	TIME	REPS	TIME	REPS	TIME	REPS

Exercise	Set 4		Set 5		Set 6	
	TIME	REPS	TIME	REPS	TIME	REPS

Week 7

Two more weeks to go until race day. Keep cranking out your sets, and really push yourself on your active rests during weeks seven and eight. The focus for this week is 50 percent power, 30 percent muscular endurance, and 20 percent strength.

Cardio and Core

Date						
Routine	Work-to-rest ratio: 60/10 sec.					
Exercise	Set 1		Set 2		Set 3	
	TIME	REPS	TIME	REPS	TIME	REPS
TRX Side Elbow Plank						
Jumping Jacks						
Floor Oblique Crunch						
Power Jacks						
	Set 4		Set 5		Set 6	
	TIME	REPS	TIME	REPS	TIME	REPS
TRX Side Elbow Plank						
Jumping Jacks						
Floor Oblique Crunch						
Power Jacks						

Date						
Routine	Work-to-rest ratio: 60/10 sec.					
Exercise	Set 1		Set 2		Set 3	
	TIME	REPS	TIME	REPS	TIME	REPS
Floor Forward Crunch						
Floor Reverse Crunch						
Floor Oblique Crunch						
Floor V Crunch (Single Leg)						
	Set 4		Set 5		Set 6	
	TIME	REPS	TIME	REPS	TIME	REPS
Floor Forward Crunch						
Floor Reverse Crunch						
Floor Oblique Crunch						
Floor V Crunch (Single Leg)						

Date						
Routine	Work-to-rest ratio: 60/10 sec.					
Exercise	Set 1		Set 2		Set 3	
	TIME	REPS	TIME	REPS	TIME	REPS
Burpees						
Power Jacks						
Plank Double Leg Lateral Hops						
Forward and Backward Jumping						
	Set 4		Set 5		Set 6	
	TIME	REPS	TIME	REPS	TIME	REPS
Burpees						
Power Jacks						
Plank Double Leg Lateral Hops						
Forward and Backward Jumping						

Date						
Routine	Work-to-rest ratio: 60/10 sec.					
Exercise	Set 1		Set 2		Set 3	
	TIME	REPS	TIME	REPS	TIME	REPS
Power Jacks						
Stability Ball Praying Mantis						
High Knees in Place						
Floor Forward Crunch						
	Set 4		Set 5		Set 6	
	TIME	REPS	TIME	REPS	TIME	REPS
Power Jacks						
Stability Ball Praying Mantis						
High Knees in Place						
Floor Forward Crunch						

Date						
Routine	Recovery Day					
Exercise	Set 1		Set 2		Set 3	
	TIME	REPS	TIME	REPS	TIME	REPS
	Set 4		Set 5		Set 6	
	TIME	REPS	TIME	REPS	TIME	REPS

Date						
Routine	Recovery Day					
Exercise	Set 1		Set 2		Set 3	
	TIME	REPS	TIME	REPS	TIME	REPS
	Set 4		Set 5		Set 6	
	TIME	REPS	TIME	REPS	TIME	REPS

Upper and Lower Body

Upper Body

Date:

Routine: Upper Body — Time-under-tension: 30 reps in 60 sec. Active rest: Burpees 30 sec. between exercises 1 and 2

Exercise	Set 1 LBS	Set 1 REPS	Set 2 LBS	Set 2 REPS	Set 3 LBS	Set 3 REPS
Dumbbell Incline Chest Press						
Dumbbell Shoulder Press						
Chin-Ups						
Triceps Dips						

Exercise	Set 4 LBS	Set 4 REPS	Set 5 LBS	Set 5 REPS	Set 6 LBS	Set 6 REPS
Dumbbell Incline Chest Press						
Dumbbell Shoulder Press						
Chin-Ups						
Triceps Dips						

Lower Body

Date:

Routine: Lower Body — Time-under-tension: 30 reps in 60 sec. Active rest: Jump Rope 30 sec. between exercises 1 and 2

Exercise	Set 1 LBS	Set 1 REPS	Set 2 LBS	Set 2 REPS	Set 3 LBS	Set 3 REPS
Dumbbell Pilates Squat						
Dumbbell Sumo Squat						
Dumbbell Back Lunges						
Dumbbell Forward Lunges						

Exercise	Set 4 LBS	Set 4 REPS	Set 5 LBS	Set 5 REPS	Set 6 LBS	Set 6 REPS
Dumbbell Pilates Squat						
Dumbbell Sumo Squat						
Dumbbell Back Lunges						
Dumbbell Forward Lunges						

Full Body

Date:

Routine: Full Body — Time-under-tension: 30 reps in 60 sec. Active rest: High Knees 30 sec. between exercises 3 and 4

Exercise	Set 1 LBS	Set 1 REPS	Set 2 LBS	Set 2 REPS	Set 3 LBS	Set 3 REPS
Dumbbell Biceps Curl						
Dumbbell Calf Raises						
Dumbbell Triceps Kick Back						
Dumbbell Back Diagonal Lunges						

Exercise	Set 4 LBS	Set 4 REPS	Set 5 LBS	Set 5 REPS	Set 6 LBS	Set 6 REPS
Dumbbell Biceps Curl						
Dumbbell Calf Raises						
Dumbbell Triceps Kick Back						
Dumbbell Back Diagonal Lunges						

Split

Date:

Routine: Split — Work-to-rest ratio: 60/10 sec. Active rest: Jumping Jacks 30 sec. between exercises 2 and 3

Exercise	Set 1 LBS	Set 1 REPS	Set 2 LBS	Set 2 REPS	Set 3 LBS	Set 3 REPS
Pull-Ups						
Dumbbell Shoulder Press						
Dumbbell Squat						
Butt Hip Raises						

Exercise	Set 4 LBS	Set 4 REPS	Set 5 LBS	Set 5 REPS	Set 6 LBS	Set 6 REPS
Pull-Ups						
Dumbbell Shoulder Press						
Dumbbell Squat						
Butt Hip Raises						

Recovery Day

Date:

Routine: Recovery Day

Recovery Day

Date:

Routine: Recovery Day

Compound and Functional

Table 1 (Column 1)

Date						
Routine	Work-to-rest ratio: 60/10 sec. Active rest: Burpees for 30 sec. between exercises 2 and 3					
Exercise	Set 1		Set 2		Set 3	
	TIME	REPS	TIME	REPS	TIME	REPS
Lateral Box Push-Offs						
Tuck Jumps						
TRX Superman						
Powerdive Push-Up						
	Set 4		Set 5		Set 6	
	TIME	REPS	TIME	REPS	TIME	REPS
Lateral Box Push-Offs						
Tuck Jumps						
TRX Superman						
Powerdive Push-Up						

Table 1 (Column 2)

Date						
Routine	Work-to-rest ratio: 60/10 sec. Active rest: Jump Rope for 30 sec. between exercises 2 and 3					
Exercise	Set 1		Set 2		Set 3	
	TIME	REPS	TIME	REPS	TIME	REPS
TRX Suspended Side Plank with Twist and Pike						
TRX Hack Squat						
TRX Atomic Push-Up						
BOSU Forward Burpee with Squat Hop-Up Onto BOSU						
	Set 4		Set 5		Set 6	
	TIME	REPS	TIME	REPS	TIME	REPS
TRX Suspended Side Plank with Twist and Pike						
TRX Hack Squat						
TRX Atomic Push-Up						
BOSU Forward Burpee with Squat Hop-Up Onto BOSU						

Table 1 (Column 3)

Date						
Routine	Work-to-rest ratio: 60/10 sec. Active rest: Jumping Jacks for 30 sec. between exercises 1 and 2					
Exercise	Set 1		Set 2		Set 3	
	TIME	REPS	TIME	REPS	TIME	REPS
Floor Bear Crawls						
Explosive Start Throws						
Lateral Jump to Box						
Lateral Hurdle Jumps						
	Set 4		Set 5		Set 6	
	TIME	REPS	TIME	REPS	TIME	REPS
Floor Bear Crawls						
Explosive Start Throws						
Lateral Jump to Box						
Lateral Hurdle Jumps						

Table 2 (Column 1)

Date						
Routine	Work-to-rest ratio: 60/10 sec. Active rest: Burpees for 30 sec. between exercises 2 and 3					
Exercise	Set 1		Set 2		Set 3	
	TIME	REPS	TIME	REPS	TIME	REPS
Circle Shoulder Raises						
TRX Tornado Twist						
TRX Suspended V Pike						
TRX Suspended Side Plank with Twist						
	Set 4		Set 5		Set 6	
	TIME	REPS	TIME	REPS	TIME	REPS
Circle Shoulder Raises						
TRX Tornado Twist						
TRX Suspended V Pike						
TRX Suspended Side Plank with Twist						

Table 2 (Column 2)

Date						
Routine	Recovery Day					
Exercise	Set 1		Set 2		Set 3	
	TIME	REPS	TIME	REPS	TIME	REPS

Table 2 (Column 3)

Date						
Routine	Recovery Day					
Exercise	Set 1		Set 2		Set 3	
	TIME	REPS	TIME	REPS	TIME	REPS

Endurance

Mon	Tue	Wed	Thu	Fri	Sat	Sun
Rest	3-mile run	8×400	3-mile run	Rest	5-mile fast	7-mile run

Week 8

Seven weeks ago you started out with a solid fitness foundation, and you've been building on it ever since. With your increased strength and endurance, you are at a competitive level. During this final week of training, begin to visualize yourself attacking the obstacles as you workout.

The final week of training puts 50 percent of the focus on muscular endurance, 30 percent on strength, and 20 percent on power.

Cardio and Core

Date							Date							Date						
Routine	Work-to-rest ratio: 60/10 sec.						Routine	Work-to-rest ratio: 60/10 sec.						Routine	Work-to-rest ratio: 60/10 sec.					
Exercise	Set 1		Set 2		Set 3		Exercise	Set 1		Set 2		Set 3		Exercise	Set 1		Set 2		Set 3	
	TIME	REPS	TIME	REPS	TIME	REPS		TIME	REPS	TIME	REPS	TIME	REPS		TIME	REPS	TIME	REPS	TIME	REPS
Stability Ball Praying Mantis							Lateral Jumping							Floor Reverse Crunch						
Floor Oblique Crunch							Forward and Backward Jumping							Mountain Climbers						
Floor Pendulum Oblique Twists							High Knees in Place							Floor Push-Up Plank						
Floor Reverse Crunch							Burpees							Forward and Backward Jumping						
	Set 4		Set 5		Set 6			Set 4		Set 5		Set 6			Set 4		Set 5		Set 6	
	TIME	REPS	TIME	REPS	TIME	REPS		TIME	REPS	TIME	REPS	TIME	REPS		TIME	REPS	TIME	REPS	TIME	REPS
Stability Ball Praying Mantis							Lateral Jumping							Floor Reverse Crunch						
Floor Oblique Crunch							Forward and Backward Jumping							Mountain Climbers						
Floor Pendulum Oblique Twists							High Knees in Place							Floor Push-Up Plank						
Floor Reverse Crunch							Burpees							Forward and Backward Jumping						

Date							Date							Date						
Routine	Work-to-rest ratio: 60/10 sec.						Routine	Recovery Day						Routine	Recovery Day					
Exercise	Set 1		Set 2		Set 3		Exercise	Set 1		Set 2		Set 3		Exercise	Set 1		Set 2		Set 3	
	TIME	REPS	TIME	REPS	TIME	REPS		TIME	REPS	TIME	REPS	TIME	REPS		TIME	REPS	TIME	REPS	TIME	REPS
Jump Rope																				
Floor Reverse Crunch																				
Plank Double Leg Lateral Hops																				
Floor Oblique Crunch																				
	Set 4		Set 5		Set 6			Set 4		Set 5		Set 6			Set 4		Set 5		Set 6	
	TIME	REPS	TIME	REPS	TIME	REPS		TIME	REPS	TIME	REPS	TIME	REPS		TIME	REPS	TIME	REPS	TIME	REPS
Jump Rope																				
Floor Reverse Crunch																				
Plank Double Leg Lateral Hops																				
Floor Oblique Crunch																				

Upper and Lower Body

Date							Date							Date						
Routine	Upper Body — Work-to-rest ratio: 60/10 sec. Active rest: High Knees 30 sec. between exercises 1 and 2						**Routine**	Lower Body — Work-to-rest ratio: 60/10 sec. Active rest: Mountain Climbers 30 sec. between exercises 2 and 3						**Routine**	Full Body — Work-to-rest ratio: 60/10 sec. Active rest: Burpees 30 sec. between exercises 2 and 3					
Exercise	Set 1		Set 2		Set 3		**Exercise**	Set 1		Set 2		Set 3		**Exercise**	Set 1		Set 2		Set 3	
	LBS	REPS	LBS	REPS	LBS	REPS		LBS	REPS	LBS	REPS	LBS	REPS		LBS	REPS	LBS	REPS	LBS	REPS
Dumbbell Triceps Overhead Extension							Dumbbell Squat							Dumbbell Back Rows						
Chin-Ups							Dumbbell Back Lunges							Dumbbell Chest Flies						
Dumbbell Chest Press							Side Lying Leg Raises							Dumbbell Sumo Squat						
Dumbbell Biceps Curl							Dumbbell Calf Raises							Dumbbell Forward Lunges						
	Set 4		Set 5		Set 6			Set 4		Set 5		Set 6			Set 4		Set 5		Set 6	
	LBS	REPS	LBS	REPS	LBS	REPS		LBS	REPS	LBS	REPS	LBS	REPS		LBS	REPS	LBS	REPS	LBS	REPS
Dumbbell Triceps Overhead Extension							Dumbbell Squat							Dumbbell Back Rows						
Chin-Ups							Dumbbell Back Lunges							Dumbbell Chest Flies						
Dumbbell Chest Press							Side Lying Leg Raises							Dumbbell Sumo Squat						
Dumbbell Biceps Curl							Dumbbell Calf Raises							Dumbbell Forward Lunges						

Date							Date							Date						
Routine	Split — Time-under-tension: 30 reps in 60 sec. Active rest: Jump Rope 30 sec. between exercises 1 and 2						**Routine**	Recovery Day						**Routine**	Recovery Day					
Exercise	Set 1		Set 2		Set 3		**Exercise**	Set 1		Set 2		Set 3		**Exercise**	Set 1		Set 2		Set 3	
	LBS	REPS	LBS	REPS	LBS	REPS		LBS	REPS	LBS	REPS	LBS	REPS		LBS	REPS	LBS	REPS	LBS	REPS
Dumbbell Shoulder Press																				
Dumbbell Pilates Squat																				
Dumbbell Deltoid Lateral Raise																				
Butt Hip Raises																				
	Set 4		Set 5		Set 6			Set 4		Set 5		Set 6			Set 4		Set 5		Set 6	
	LBS	REPS	LBS	REPS	LBS	REPS		LBS	REPS	LBS	REPS	LBS	REPS		LBS	REPS	LBS	REPS	LBS	REPS
Dumbbell Shoulder Press																				
Dumbbell Pilates Squat																				
Dumbbell Deltoid Lateral Raise																				
Butt Hip Raises																				

Compound and Functional

Routine 1

Date

Routine: Work-to-rest ratio: 60/10 sec. Active rest: Burpees for 30 sec. between exercises 2 and 3

Exercise	Set 1 TIME	Set 1 REPS	Set 2 TIME	Set 2 REPS	Set 3 TIME	Set 3 REPS
TRX Atomic Push-Up						
TRX Hack Squat						
Circle Shoulder Raises						
TRX Seated Pull-Up						

Exercise	Set 4 TIME	Set 4 REPS	Set 5 TIME	Set 5 REPS	Set 6 TIME	Set 6 REPS
TRX Atomic Push-Up						
TRX Hack Squat						
Circle Shoulder Raises						
TRX Seated Pull-Up						

Routine 2

Date

Routine: Work-to-rest ratio: 60/10 sec. Active rest: Floor Bear Crawls for 30 sec. between exercises 1 and 2

Exercise	Set 1 TIME	Set 1 REPS	Set 2 TIME	Set 2 REPS	Set 3 TIME	Set 3 REPS
Squat Throws						
TRX Suspended Side Plank with Twist						
Diagonal Forward Bounding						
BOSU Balance Trainer High Knees with One Leg On and One Leg Off						

Exercise	Set 4 TIME	Set 4 REPS	Set 5 TIME	Set 5 REPS	Set 6 TIME	Set 6 REPS
Squat Throws						
TRX Suspended Side Plank with Twist						
Diagonal Forward Bounding						
BOSU Balance Trainer High Knees with One Leg On and One Leg Off						

Routine 3

Date

Routine: Work-to-rest ratio: 60/10 sec. Active rest: High Knees for 30 sec. between exercises 1 and 2

Exercise	Set 1 TIME	Set 1 REPS	Set 2 TIME	Set 2 REPS	Set 3 TIME	Set 3 REPS
Lateral Box Push-Offs						
TRX Suspended Walking Plank						
TRX Seated Pull-Up						
BOSU Reverse Burpee and Roll-Up Squat Hop-Up						

Exercise	Set 4 TIME	Set 4 REPS	Set 5 TIME	Set 5 REPS	Set 6 TIME	Set 6 REPS
Lateral Box Push-Offs						
TRX Suspended Walking Plank						
TRX Seated Pull-Up						
BOSU Reverse Burpee and Roll-Up Squat Hop-Up						

Routine 4

Date

Routine: Work-to-rest ratio: 60/10 sec. Active rest: Mountain Climbers for 30 sec. between exercises 2 and 3

Exercise	Set 1 TIME	Set 1 REPS	Set 2 TIME	Set 2 REPS	Set 3 TIME	Set 3 REPS
TRX Superman						
BOSU Forward Burpee with Squat Hop-Up Onto BOSU						
Powerdive Push-Up						
Floor Bear Crawls						

Exercise	Set 4 TIME	Set 4 REPS	Set 5 TIME	Set 5 REPS	Set 6 TIME	Set 6 REPS
TRX Superman						
BOSU Forward Burpee with Squat Hop-Up Onto BOSU						
Powerdive Push-Up						
Floor Bear Crawls						

Routine 5

Date

Routine: Recovery Day

Routine 6

Date

Routine: Recovery Day

Endurance

Mon	Tue	Wed	Thu	Fri	Sat	Sun
Rest	2-mile run	30 min. tempo	2-mile run	Rest	Rest	5k race

Advanced

Your advanced level of fitness already puts you near the front of the pack for most obstacle races. After eight weeks of specialized training, you're going to be able to conquer any course.

Your total training time is 60 minutes (excluding warm-up and endurance training), five days a week. Each day focuses on a different part of your body. Days are broken down as follows:

Day 1—Upper Body:

- Dynamic warm-up (5 minutes)
- Strength training (15 minutes)
- Functional/compound training (15 minutes)
- Cardio training (15 minutes)
- Core training (10 minutes)
- Flexibility (5 minutes)

Day 2—Lower Body:

- Dynamic warm-up (5 minutes)
- Strength training (15 minutes)
- Functional/compound training (15 minutes)
- Cardio training (15 minutes)
- Core training (10 minutes)
- Flexibility (5 minutes)

Day 3—Full Body:

- Dynamic warm-up (5 minutes)
- Strength training (15 minutes)
- Functional/compound training (25 minutes)
- Cardio training (10 minutes)
- Core training (5 minutes)
- Flexibility (5 minutes)

Days 4 and 5—Split Training:

- Dynamic warm-up (5 minutes)
- Strength training (15 minutes)
- Functional/compound training (15 minutes)
- Cardio training (15 minutes)
- Core training (10 minutes)
- Flexibility (5 minutes)

Week 1

During your first and second weeks of training, you perform four sets of each exercise, working twice as long as you rest between each set. In addition, once during each day's workout, you're going to do an active rest. During an active rest, you rest the specific muscles that you just worked, but otherwise remain active by doing cardio exercises such as jumping jacks, jumping rope, or burpees for the duration of your "rest" period. These minicardio sessions are great little tools for taking your endurance and cardiovascular capacity to the next level—without adding time to your total workout. The specific active rest activity is indicated in the *Routine* section of the training sheet.

The training goals for this week's workout are as follows: 50 percent neurological adaptation, 30 percent strength, 20 percent power.

Cardio and Core

Date							Date							Date						
Routine	Work-to-rest ratio: 60/30 sec.						Routine	Work-to-rest ratio: 60/30 sec.						Routine	Work-to-rest ratio: 60/30 sec.					
Exercise	Set 1		Set 2		Set 3		Exercise	Set 1		Set 2		Set 3		Exercise	Set 1		Set 2		Set 3	
	TIME	REPS	TIME	REPS	TIME	REPS		TIME	REPS	TIME	REPS	TIME	REPS		TIME	REPS	TIME	REPS	TIME	REPS
Floor Oblique Crunch							Floor Pendulum Oblique Twists							Stability Ball Praying Mantis						
Jumping Jacks							Floor Forward Crunch							Floor V Crunch (Single Leg)						
Floor Push-Up Plank							Plank Lateral Jacks							TRX Side Elbow Plank						
Power Jacks							Jump Rope							Stability Ball Forward Crunch						
	Set 4		Set 5		Set 6			Set 4		Set 5		Set 6			Set 4		Set 5		Set 6	
	TIME	REPS	TIME	REPS	TIME	REPS		TIME	REPS	TIME	REPS	TIME	REPS		TIME	REPS	TIME	REPS	TIME	REPS
Floor Oblique Crunch							Floor Pendulum Oblique Twists							Stability Ball Praying Mantis						
Jumping Jacks							Floor Forward Crunch							Floor V Crunch (Single Leg)						
Floor Push-Up Plank							Plank Lateral Jacks							TRX Side Elbow Plank						
Power Jacks							Jump Rope							Stability Ball Forward Crunch						

Date							Date							Date						
Routine	Work-to-rest ratio: 60/30 sec.						Routine	Work-to-rest ratio: 60/30 sec.						Routine	Recovery Day					
Exercise	Set 1		Set 2		Set 3		Exercise	Set 1		Set 2		Set 3		Exercise	Set 1		Set 2		Set 3	
	TIME	REPS	TIME	REPS	TIME	REPS		TIME	REPS	TIME	REPS	TIME	REPS		TIME	REPS	TIME	REPS	TIME	REPS
Jump Rope							TRX Side Elbow Plank													
Forward and Backward Jumping							Jumping Jacks													
Lateral Jumping							Stability Ball Praying Mantis													
High Knees in Place							Power Jacks													
	Set 4		Set 5		Set 6			Set 4		Set 5		Set 6			Set 4		Set 5		Set 6	
	TIME	REPS	TIME	REPS	TIME	REPS		TIME	REPS	TIME	REPS	TIME	REPS		TIME	REPS	TIME	REPS	TIME	REPS
Jump Rope							TRX Side Elbow Plank													
Forward and Backward Jumping							Jumping Jacks													
Lateral Jumping							Stability Ball Praying Mantis													
High Knees in Place							Power Jacks													

Upper and Lower Body

Upper Body

Date						
Routine	Upper Body Time-under-tension: 15 reps in 60 sec. Active rest: Jump Rope 30 sec. between exercises 3 and 4					

Exercise	Set 1		Set 2		Set 3	
	LBS	REPS	LBS	REPS	LBS	REPS
Dumbbell Chest Press						
Dumbbell Chest Flies						
Dumbbell Back Flies						
Dumbbell Back Rows						

	Set 4		Set 5		Set 6	
	LBS	REPS	LBS	REPS	LBS	REPS
Dumbbell Chest Press						
Dumbbell Chest Flies						
Dumbbell Back Flies						
Dumbbell Back Rows						

Lower Body

Date						
Routine	Lower Body Time-under-tension: 15 reps in 60 sec. Active rest: Jumping Jacks 30 sec. between exercises 1 and 2					

Exercise	Set 1		Set 2		Set 3	
	LBS	REPS	LBS	REPS	LBS	REPS
Dumbbell Squat						
Dumbbell Back Lunges						
Side Lying Leg Raises						
Butt Hip Raises						

	Set 4		Set 5		Set 6	
	LBS	REPS	LBS	REPS	LBS	REPS
Dumbbell Squat						
Dumbbell Back Lunges						
Side Lying Leg Raises						
Butt Hip Raises						

Full Body

Date						
Routine	Full Body Time-under-tension: 15 reps in 60 sec. Active rest: High Knees 30 sec. between exercises 2 and 3					

Exercise	Set 1		Set 2		Set 3	
	LBS	REPS	LBS	REPS	LBS	REPS
Dumbbell Incline Chest Press						
Dumbbell Sumo Squat						
Dumbbell Shoulder Press						
Dumbbell Incline Biceps Curl						

	Set 4		Set 5		Set 6	
	LBS	REPS	LBS	REPS	LBS	REPS
Dumbbell Incline Chest Press						
Dumbbell Sumo Squat						
Dumbbell Shoulder Press						
Dumbbell Incline Biceps Curl						

Split

Date						
Routine	Split Work-to-rest ratio: 60/30 sec. Active rest: Jump Rope 30 sec. between exercises 1 and 2					

Exercise	Set 1		Set 2		Set 3	
	LBS	REPS	LBS	REPS	LBS	REPS
Dumbbell Chest Flies						
Dumbbell Biceps Curl						
Pull-Ups						
Chin-Ups						

	Set 4		Set 5		Set 6	
	LBS	REPS	LBS	REPS	LBS	REPS
Dumbbell Chest Flies						
Dumbbell Biceps Curl						
Pull-Ups						
Chin-Ups						

Split

Date						
Routine	Split Work-to-rest ratio: 60/30 sec. Active rest: Mountain Climbers 30 sec. between exercises 1 and 2					

Exercise	Set 1		Set 2		Set 3	
	LBS	REPS	LBS	REPS	LBS	REPS
Dumbbell Back Flies						
Chest Dips						
Dumbbell Pilates Squat						
Dumbbell Shoulder Press						

	Set 4		Set 5		Set 6	
	LBS	REPS	LBS	REPS	LBS	REPS
Dumbbell Back Flies						
Chest Dips						
Dumbbell Pilates Squat						
Dumbbell Shoulder Press						

Recovery Day

Date						
Routine	Recovery Day					

Exercise	Set 1		Set 2		Set 3	
	LBS	REPS	LBS	REPS	LBS	REPS

	Set 4		Set 5		Set 6	
	LBS	REPS	LBS	REPS	LBS	REPS

Compound and Functional

Date: _____ **Routine:** _____
Work-to-rest ratio: 60/30 sec. Active rest: Burpees for 30 sec. between exercises 2 and 3

Exercise	Set 1 TIME	Set 1 REPS	Set 2 TIME	Set 2 REPS	Set 3 TIME	Set 3 REPS
TRX Hack Squat						
Lateral Hurdle Jumps						
Powerdive Push-Up						
TRX Seated Pull-Up						

Exercise	Set 4 TIME	Set 4 REPS	Set 5 TIME	Set 5 REPS	Set 6 TIME	Set 6 REPS
TRX Hack Squat						
Lateral Hurdle Jumps						
Powerdive Push-Up						
TRX Seated Pull-Up						

Date: _____ **Routine:** _____
Work-to-rest ratio: 60/30 sec. Active rest: Jump Rope for 30 sec. between exercises 2 and 3

Exercise	Set 1 TIME	Set 1 REPS	Set 2 TIME	Set 2 REPS	Set 3 TIME	Set 3 REPS
Forward Hurdle Running						
Sideways Hurdle Running						
Floor Bear Crawls						
Tuck Jumps						

Exercise	Set 4 TIME	Set 4 REPS	Set 5 TIME	Set 5 REPS	Set 6 TIME	Set 6 REPS
Forward Hurdle Running						
Sideways Hurdle Running						
Floor Bear Crawls						
Tuck Jumps						

Date: _____ **Routine:** _____
Work-to-rest ratio: 60/30 sec. Active rest: Jumping Jacks for 30 sec. between exercises 1 and 2

Exercise	Set 1 TIME	Set 1 REPS	Set 2 TIME	Set 2 REPS	Set 3 TIME	Set 3 REPS
TRX Suspended Leg Circles						
TRX Suspended V Pike						
TRX Suspended Side Plank with Twist and Pike						
TRX Suspended Side Plank with Twist						

Exercise	Set 4 TIME	Set 4 REPS	Set 5 TIME	Set 5 REPS	Set 6 TIME	Set 6 REPS
TRX Suspended Leg Circles						
TRX Suspended V Pike						
TRX Suspended Side Plank with Twist and Pike						
TRX Suspended Side Plank with Twist						

Date: _____ **Routine:** _____
Work-to-rest ratio: 60/30 sec. Active rest: Burpees for 30 sec. between exercises 2 and 3

Exercise	Set 1 TIME	Set 1 REPS	Set 2 TIME	Set 2 REPS	Set 3 TIME	Set 3 REPS
Lateral Hurdle Jumps						
Lateral Jump to Box						
TRX Superman						
Diagonal Forward Bounding						

Exercise	Set 4 TIME	Set 4 REPS	Set 5 TIME	Set 5 REPS	Set 6 TIME	Set 6 REPS
Lateral Hurdle Jumps						
Lateral Jump to Box						
TRX Superman						
Diagonal Forward Bounding						

Date: _____ **Routine:** _____
Work-to-rest ratio: 60/30 sec. Active rest: High Knees for 30 sec. between exercises 2 and 3

Exercise	Set 1 TIME	Set 1 REPS	Set 2 TIME	Set 2 REPS	Set 3 TIME	Set 3 REPS
TRX Atomic Push-Up						
BOSU Balance Trainer High Knees with One Leg On and One Leg Off						
Explosive Start Throws						
Squat Throws						

Exercise	Set 4 TIME	Set 4 REPS	Set 5 TIME	Set 5 REPS	Set 6 TIME	Set 6 REPS
TRX Atomic Push-Up						
BOSU Balance Trainer High Knees with One Leg On and One Leg Off						
Explosive Start Throws						
Squat Throws						

Date: _____ **Routine:** _____
Recovery Day

Endurance

Mon	Tue	Wed	Thu	Fri	Sat	Sun
3-mile run	5×400	Rest or easy run	30 min. tempo	Rest	4-mile fast	60 min. run

Week 2

During week two, continue performing four sets of each exercise. This week's workout emphasizes 50 percent strength, 30 percent power, and 20 percent neurological adaptation.

Cardio and Core

Date							Date							Date						
Routine	Work-to-rest ratio: 60/30 sec.						Routine	Work-to-rest ratio: 60/30 sec.						Routine	Work-to-rest ratio: 60/30 sec.					
Exercise	Set 1		Set 2		Set 3		Exercise	Set 1		Set 2		Set 3		Exercise	Set 1		Set 2		Set 3	
	TIME	REPS	TIME	REPS	TIME	REPS		TIME	REPS	TIME	REPS	TIME	REPS		TIME	REPS	TIME	REPS	TIME	REPS
Jumping Jacks							Plank Lateral Jacks							Floor Push-Up Plank						
Stability Ball Praying Mantis							Floor Oblique Crunch							Floor Reverse Crunch						
Burpees							Floor Pendulum Oblique Twists							Mountain Climbers						
Floor Oblique Crunch							Lateral Jumping							Stability Ball Forward Crunch						
	Set 4		Set 5		Set 6			Set 4		Set 5		Set 6			Set 4		Set 5		Set 6	
	TIME	REPS	TIME	REPS	TIME	REPS		TIME	REPS	TIME	REPS	TIME	REPS		TIME	REPS	TIME	REPS	TIME	REPS
Jumping Jacks							Plank Lateral Jacks							Floor Push-Up Plank						
Stability Ball Praying Mantis							Floor Oblique Crunch							Floor Reverse Crunch						
Burpees							Floor Pendulum Oblique Twists							Mountain Climbers						
Floor Oblique Crunch							Lateral Jumping							Stability Ball Forward Crunch						

Date							Date							Date						
Routine	Work-to-rest ratio: 60/30 sec.						Routine	Work-to-rest ratio: 60/30 sec.						Routine	Recovery Day					
Exercise	Set 1		Set 2		Set 3		Exercise	Set 1		Set 2		Set 3		Exercise	Set 1		Set 2		Set 3	
	TIME	REPS	TIME	REPS	TIME	REPS		TIME	REPS	TIME	REPS	TIME	REPS		TIME	REPS	TIME	REPS	TIME	REPS
Floor Forward Crunch							Floor Reverse Crunch													
Floor Reverse Crunch							Floor Push-Up Plank													
Jump Rope							Stability Ball Praying Mantis													
Power Jacks							Plank Lateral Jacks													
	Set 4		Set 5		Set 6			Set 4		Set 5		Set 6			Set 4		Set 5		Set 6	
	TIME	REPS	TIME	REPS	TIME	REPS		TIME	REPS	TIME	REPS	TIME	REPS		TIME	REPS	TIME	REPS	TIME	REPS
Floor Forward Crunch							Floor Reverse Crunch													
Floor Reverse Crunch							Floor Push-Up Plank													
Jump Rope							Stability Ball Praying Mantis													
Power Jacks							Plank Lateral Jacks													

Upper and Lower Body

Upper Body

Date:

Routine: Upper Body
Work-to-rest ratio 60/30 sec.
Active rest: Jump Rope 30 sec. between exercises 2 and 3

Exercise	Set 1 LBS	Set 1 REPS	Set 2 LBS	Set 2 REPS	Set 3 LBS	Set 3 REPS
Dumbbell Shoulder Press						
Dumbbell Incline Chest Press						
Triceps Dips						
Chin-Ups						

Exercise	Set 4 LBS	Set 4 REPS	Set 5 LBS	Set 5 REPS	Set 6 LBS	Set 6 REPS
Dumbbell Shoulder Press						
Dumbbell Incline Chest Press						
Triceps Dips						
Chin-Ups						

Lower Body

Date:

Routine: Lower Body
Work-to-rest ratio: 60/30 sec.
Active rest: Jumping Jacks 30 sec. between exercises 3 and 4

Exercise	Set 1 LBS	Set 1 REPS	Set 2 LBS	Set 2 REPS	Set 3 LBS	Set 3 REPS
Butt Hip Raises						
Dumbbell Squat						
Dumbbell Calf Raises						
Dumbbell Back Diagonal Lunges						

Exercise	Set 4 LBS	Set 4 REPS	Set 5 LBS	Set 5 REPS	Set 6 LBS	Set 6 REPS
Butt Hip Raises						
Dumbbell Squat						
Dumbbell Calf Raises						
Dumbbell Back Diagonal Lunges						

Full Body

Date:

Routine: Full Body
Work-to-rest ratio: 60/30 sec.
Active rest: High Knees 30 sec. between exercises 2 and 3

Exercise	Set 1 LBS	Set 1 REPS	Set 2 LBS	Set 2 REPS	Set 3 LBS	Set 3 REPS
Dumbbell Chest Press						
Pull-Ups						
Dumbbell Triceps Kick Back						
Dumbbell Back Rows						

Exercise	Set 4 LBS	Set 4 REPS	Set 5 LBS	Set 5 REPS	Set 6 LBS	Set 6 REPS
Dumbbell Chest Press						
Pull-Ups						
Dumbbell Triceps Kick Back						
Dumbbell Back Rows						

Split

Date:

Routine: Split
Time-under-tension: 15 reps in 60 sec.
Active rest: Jump Rope 30 sec. between exercises 2 and 3

Exercise	Set 1 LBS	Set 1 REPS	Set 2 LBS	Set 2 REPS	Set 3 LBS	Set 3 REPS
Dumbbell Back Rows						
Dumbbell Back Diagonal Lunges						
Dumbbell Shoulder Press						
Butt Hip Raises						

Exercise	Set 4 LBS	Set 4 REPS	Set 5 LBS	Set 5 REPS	Set 6 LBS	Set 6 REPS
Dumbbell Back Rows						
Dumbbell Back Diagonal Lunges						
Dumbbell Shoulder Press						
Butt Hip Raises						

Split

Date:

Routine: Split
Time-under-tension: 15 reps in 60 sec.
Active rest: High Knees 30 sec. between exercises 2 and 3

Exercise	Set 1 LBS	Set 1 REPS	Set 2 LBS	Set 2 REPS	Set 3 LBS	Set 3 REPS
Dumbbell Squat						
Dumbbell Biceps Curl						
Triceps Dips						
Dumbbell Forward Lunges						

Exercise	Set 4 LBS	Set 4 REPS	Set 5 LBS	Set 5 REPS	Set 6 LBS	Set 6 REPS
Dumbbell Squat						
Dumbbell Biceps Curl						
Triceps Dips						
Dumbbell Forward Lunges						

Recovery Day

Date:

Routine: Recovery Day

Exercise	Set 1 LBS	Set 1 REPS	Set 2 LBS	Set 2 REPS	Set 3 LBS	Set 3 REPS

Exercise	Set 4 LBS	Set 4 REPS	Set 5 LBS	Set 5 REPS	Set 6 LBS	Set 6 REPS

Compound and Functional

Block 1

Date						
Routine	Work-to-rest ratio: 60/30 sec. Active rest: Burpees for 30 sec. between exercises 2 and 3					
Exercise	Set 1		Set 2		Set 3	
	TIME	REPS	TIME	REPS	TIME	REPS
TRX Hack Squat						
Lateral Box Push-Offs						
Powerdive Push-Up						
TRX Seated Pull-Up						
	Set 4		Set 5		Set 6	
	TIME	REPS	TIME	REPS	TIME	REPS
TRX Hack Squat						
Lateral Box Push-Offs						
Powerdive Push-Up						
TRX Seated Pull-Up						

Block 2

Date						
Routine	Work-to-rest ratio: 60/30 sec. Active rest: Floor Bear Crawls for 30 sec. between exercises 1 and 2					
Exercise	Set 1		Set 2		Set 3	
	TIME	REPS	TIME	REPS	TIME	REPS
Forward Hurdle Running						
Sideways Hurdle Running						
Floor Bear Crawls						
Tuck Jumps						
	Set 4		Set 5		Set 6	
	TIME	REPS	TIME	REPS	TIME	REPS
Forward Hurdle Running						
Sideways Hurdle Running						
Floor Bear Crawls						
Tuck Jumps						

Block 3

Date						
Routine	Work-to-rest ratio: 60/30 sec. Active rest: Jump Rope for 30 sec. between exercises 1 and 2					
Exercise	Set 1		Set 2		Set 3	
	TIME	REPS	TIME	REPS	TIME	REPS
TRX Suspended Leg Circles						
TRX Suspended V Pike						
TRX Suspended Side Plank with Twist and Pike						
TRX Suspended Side Plank with Twist						
	Set 4		Set 5		Set 6	
	TIME	REPS	TIME	REPS	TIME	REPS
TRX Suspended Leg Circles						
TRX Suspended V Pike						
TRX Suspended Side Plank with Twist and Pike						
TRX Suspended Side Plank with Twist						

Block 4

Date						
Routine	Work-to-rest ratio: 60/30 sec. Active rest: Mountain Climbers for 30 sec. between exercises 2 and 3					
Exercise	Set 1		Set 2		Set 3	
	TIME	REPS	TIME	REPS	TIME	REPS
Lateral Hurdle Jumps						
Lateral Jump to Box						
TRX Superman						
Diagonal Forward Bounding						
	Set 4		Set 5		Set 6	
	TIME	REPS	TIME	REPS	TIME	REPS
Lateral Hurdle Jumps						
Lateral Jump to Box						
TRX Superman						
Diagonal Forward Bounding						

Block 5

Date						
Routine	Work-to-rest ratio: 60/30 sec. Active rest: Mountain Climbers for 30 sec. between exercises 2 and 3					
Exercise	Set 1		Set 2		Set 3	
	TIME	REPS	TIME	REPS	TIME	REPS
TRX Atomic Push-Up						
BOSU Balance Trainer High Knees with One Leg On and One Leg Off						
Explosive Start Throws						
Squat Throws						
	Set 4		Set 5		Set 6	
	TIME	REPS	TIME	REPS	TIME	REPS
TRX Atomic Push-Up						
BOSU Balance Trainer High Knees with One Leg On and One Leg Off						
Explosive Start Throws						
Squat Throws						

Block 6

Date						
Routine	Recovery Day					
Exercise	Set 1		Set 2		Set 3	
	TIME	REPS	TIME	REPS	TIME	REPS
	Set 4		Set 5		Set 6	
	TIME	REPS	TIME	REPS	TIME	REPS

Endurance

Mon	Tue	Wed	Thu	Fri	Sat	Sun
3-mile run	8×200	Rest or easy run	30 min. tempo	Rest	4-mile fast	65 min. run

Week 3

Now that you have two weeks of training under your belt, you're going to up the number of sets to five, and decrease the rest time between each set. During week three, continue performing an active rest exercise once during each workout. The workout goals this week are 50 percent power, 30 percent muscular endurance, and 20 percent strength.

Cardio and Core

Date							Date							Date						
Routine	Work-to-rest ratio: 60/30 sec.						Routine	Work-to-rest ratio: 60/30 sec.						Routine	Work-to-rest ratio: 60/30 sec.					
Exercise	Set 1		Set 2		Set 3		Exercise	Set 1		Set 2		Set 3		Exercise	Set 1		Set 2		Set 3	
	TIME	REPS	TIME	REPS	TIME	REPS		TIME	REPS	TIME	REPS	TIME	REPS		TIME	REPS	TIME	REPS	TIME	REPS
Floor Push-Up Plank							Forward and Backward Jumping							TRX Side Elbow Plank						
Floor V Crunch (Single Leg)							Power Jacks							High Knees in Place						
Floor Reverse Crunch							Jump Rope							Floor Pendulum Oblique Twists						
Floor Forward Crunch							Lateral Jumping							Forward and Backward Jumping						
	Set 4		Set 5		Set 6			Set 4		Set 5		Set 6			Set 4		Set 5		Set 6	
	TIME	REPS	TIME	REPS	TIME	REPS		TIME	REPS	TIME	REPS	TIME	REPS		TIME	REPS	TIME	REPS	TIME	REPS
Floor Push-Up Plank							Forward and Backward Jumping							TRX Side Elbow Plank						
Floor V Crunch (Single Leg)							Power Jacks							High Knees in Place						
Floor Reverse Crunch							Jump Rope							Floor Pendulum Oblique Twists						
Floor Forward Crunch							Lateral Jumping							Forward and Backward Jumping						

Date							Date							Date						
Routine	Work-to-rest ratio: 60/30 sec.						Routine	Work-to-rest ratio: 60/30 sec.						Routine	Recovery Day					
Exercise	Set 1		Set 2		Set 3		Exercise	Set 1		Set 2		Set 3		Exercise	Set 1		Set 2		Set 3	
	TIME	REPS	TIME	REPS	TIME	REPS		TIME	REPS	TIME	REPS	TIME	REPS		TIME	REPS	TIME	REPS	TIME	REPS
Stability Ball Forward Crunch							Forward and Backward Jumping													
Floor V Crunch (Single Leg)							Jumping Jacks													
Power Jacks							Stability Ball Forward Crunch													
Lateral Jumping							Floor Pendulum Oblique Twists													
	Set 4		Set 5		Set 6			Set 4		Set 5		Set 6			Set 4		Set 5		Set 6	
	TIME	REPS	TIME	REPS	TIME	REPS		TIME	REPS	TIME	REPS	TIME	REPS		TIME	REPS	TIME	REPS	TIME	REPS
Stability Ball Forward Crunch							Forward and Backward Jumping													
Floor V Crunch (Single Leg)							Jumping Jacks													
Power Jacks							Stability Ball Forward Crunch													
Lateral Jumping							Floor Pendulum Oblique Twists													

Upper and Lower Body

Date							Date							Date						
Routine	Upper Body. Time-under-tension: 20 reps in 60 sec. Active rest: Jump Rope 30 sec. between exercises 1 and 2						**Routine**	Lower Body. Time-under-tension: 20 reps in 60 sec. Active rest: Jumping Jacks 30 sec. between exercises 1 and 2						**Routine**	Full Body. Time-under-tension: 20 reps in 60 sec. Active rest: High Knees 30 sec. between exercises 3 and 4					
Exercise	Set 1		Set 2		Set 3		**Exercise**	Set 1		Set 2		Set 3		**Exercise**	Set 1		Set 2		Set 3	
	LBS	REPS	LBS	REPS	LBS	REPS		LBS	REPS	LBS	REPS	LBS	REPS		LBS	REPS	LBS	REPS	LBS	REPS
Dumbbell Triceps Kick Back							Dumbbell Pilates Squat							Dumbbell Chest Flies						
Dumbbell Incline Chest Press							Side Lying Leg Raises							Dumbbell Squat						
Dumbbell Shoulder Press							Dumbbell Back Lunges							Dumbbell Back Flies						
Chin-Ups							Butt Hip Raises							Dumbbell Back Diagonal Lunges						
	Set 4		Set 5		Set 6			Set 4		Set 5		Set 6			Set 4		Set 5		Set 6	
	LBS	REPS	LBS	REPS	LBS	REPS		LBS	REPS	LBS	REPS	LBS	REPS		LBS	REPS	LBS	REPS	LBS	REPS
Dumbbell Triceps Kick Back							Dumbbell Pilates Squat							Dumbbell Chest Flies						
Dumbbell Incline Chest Press							Side Lying Leg Raises							Dumbbell Squat						
Dumbbell Shoulder Press							Dumbbell Back Lunges							Dumbbell Back Flies						
Chin-Ups							Butt Hip Raises							Dumbbell Back Diagonal Lunges						

Date							Date							Date						
Routine	Split. Work-to-rest ratio: 60/20 sec. Active rest: Jump Rope 30 sec. between exercises 2 and 3						**Routine**	Split. Work-to-rest ratio: 60/20 sec. Active rest: Jump Rope 30 sec. between exercises 2 and 3						**Routine**	Recovery Day					
Exercise	Set 1		Set 2		Set 3		**Exercise**	Set 1		Set 2		Set 3		**Exercise**	Set 1		Set 2		Set 3	
	LBS	REPS	LBS	REPS	LBS	REPS		LBS	REPS	LBS	REPS	LBS	REPS		LBS	REPS	LBS	REPS	LBS	REPS
Dumbbell Chest Flies							Dumbbell Pilates Squat													
Dumbbell Back Flies							Side Lying Leg Raises													
Side Lying Leg Raises							Dumbbell Chest Flies													
Butt Hip Raises							Dumbbell Back Rows													
	Set 4		Set 5		Set 6			Set 4		Set 5		Set 6			Set 4		Set 5		Set 6	
	LBS	REPS	LBS	REPS	LBS	REPS		LBS	REPS	LBS	REPS	LBS	REPS		LBS	REPS	LBS	REPS	LBS	REPS
Dumbbell Chest Flies							Dumbbell Pilates Squat													
Dumbbell Back Flies							Side Lying Leg Raises													
Side Lying Leg Raises							Dumbbell Chest Flies													
Butt Hip Raises							Dumbbell Back Rows													

Compound and Functional

Block 1

Date: _____
Routine: Work-to-rest ratio: 60/20 sec. Active rest: Burpees for 30 sec. between exercises 2 and 3

Exercise	Set 1 TIME	Set 1 REPS	Set 2 TIME	Set 2 REPS	Set 3 TIME	Set 3 REPS	Set 4 TIME	Set 4 REPS	Set 5 TIME	Set 5 REPS	Set 6 TIME	Set 6 REPS
Circle Shoulder Raises												
TRX Hack Squat												
Circle Shoulder Raises												
TRX Atomic Push-Up												

Block 2

Date: _____
Routine: Work-to-rest ratio: 60/20 sec. Active rest: Jump Rope for 30 sec. between exercises 2 and 3

Exercise	Set 1 TIME	Set 1 REPS	Set 2 TIME	Set 2 REPS	Set 3 TIME	Set 3 REPS	Set 4 TIME	Set 4 REPS	Set 5 TIME	Set 5 REPS	Set 6 TIME	Set 6 REPS
BOSU Forward Burpee with Squat Hop-Up Onto BOSU												
TRX Seated Pull-Up												
TRX Superman												
TRX Atomic Push-Up												

Block 3

Date: _____
Routine: Work-to-rest ratio: 60/20 sec. Active rest: Jumping Jacks for 30 sec. between exercises 1 and 2

Exercise	Set 1 TIME	Set 1 REPS	Set 2 TIME	Set 2 REPS	Set 3 TIME	Set 3 REPS	Set 4 TIME	Set 4 REPS	Set 5 TIME	Set 5 REPS	Set 6 TIME	Set 6 REPS
TRX Suspended Leg Circles												
TRX Suspended Walking Plank												
Lateral Box Push-Offs												
Squat Throws												

Block 4

Date: _____
Routine: Work-to-rest ratio: 60/20 sec. Active rest: Burpees for 30 sec. between exercises 2 and 3

Exercise	Set 1 TIME	Set 1 REPS	Set 2 TIME	Set 2 REPS	Set 3 TIME	Set 3 REPS	Set 4 TIME	Set 4 REPS	Set 5 TIME	Set 5 REPS	Set 6 TIME	Set 6 REPS
Forward Hurdle Running												
Floor Bear Crawls												
Diagonal Forward Bounding												
Powerdive Push-Up												

Block 5

Date: _____
Routine: Work-to-rest ratio: 60/20 sec. Active rest: Burpees for 30 sec. between exercises 2 and 3

Exercise	Set 1 TIME	Set 1 REPS	Set 2 TIME	Set 2 REPS	Set 3 TIME	Set 3 REPS	Set 4 TIME	Set 4 REPS	Set 5 TIME	Set 5 REPS	Set 6 TIME	Set 6 REPS
Your Choice												
Your Choice												
Your Choice												
Your Choice												

Block 6

Date: _____
Routine: Recovery Day

Exercise	Set 1 TIME	Set 1 REPS	Set 2 TIME	Set 2 REPS	Set 3 TIME	Set 3 REPS	Set 4 TIME	Set 4 REPS	Set 5 TIME	Set 5 REPS	Set 6 TIME	Set 6 REPS

Endurance

Mon	Tue	Wed	Thu	Fri	Sat	Sun
3-mile run	6×400	Rest or easy run	35 min. tempo	Rest	5-mile fast	70 min. run

Week 4

With three weeks of training under your belt, you should be feeling stronger and more energized during each training session in week four. If you're combining your workout with a healthy diet, you've probably also shed a few pounds and are feeling lean, mean, and ready to take on the course.

The training goals for this week are as follows: 50 percent strength, 30 percent muscular endurance, 20 percent power.

Cardio and Core

Date:
Routine: Work-to-rest ratio: 60/20 sec.

Exercise	Set 1 TIME	Set 1 REPS	Set 2 TIME	Set 2 REPS	Set 3 TIME	Set 3 REPS
Stability Ball Praying Mantis						
Jump Rope						
Floor Reverse Crunch						
Forward and Backward Jumping						

Exercise	Set 4 TIME	Set 4 REPS	Set 5 TIME	Set 5 REPS	Set 6 TIME	Set 6 REPS
Stability Ball Praying Mantis						
Jump Rope						
Floor Reverse Crunch						
Forward and Backward Jumping						

Date:
Routine: Work-to-rest ratio: 60/20 sec.

Exercise	Set 1 TIME	Set 1 REPS	Set 2 TIME	Set 2 REPS	Set 3 TIME	Set 3 REPS
Floor Oblique Crunch						
Burpees						
Floor Push-Up Plank						
Lateral Jumping						

Exercise	Set 4 TIME	Set 4 REPS	Set 5 TIME	Set 5 REPS	Set 6 TIME	Set 6 REPS
Floor Oblique Crunch						
Burpees						
Floor Push-Up Plank						
Lateral Jumping						

Date:
Routine: Work-to-rest ratio: 60/20 sec.

Exercise	Set 1 TIME	Set 1 REPS	Set 2 TIME	Set 2 REPS	Set 3 TIME	Set 3 REPS
Floor Forward Crunch						
High Knees in Place						
Mountain Climbers						
Floor V Crunch (Single Leg)						

Exercise	Set 4 TIME	Set 4 REPS	Set 5 TIME	Set 5 REPS	Set 6 TIME	Set 6 REPS
Floor Forward Crunch						
High Knees in Place						
Mountain Climbers						
Floor V Crunch (Single Leg)						

Date:
Routine: Work-to-rest ratio: 60/20 sec.

Exercise	Set 1 TIME	Set 1 REPS	Set 2 TIME	Set 2 REPS	Set 3 TIME	Set 3 REPS
Plank Double Leg Lateral Hops						
Floor Pendulum Oblique Twists						
Jump Rope						
Floor Push-Up Plank						

Exercise	Set 4 TIME	Set 4 REPS	Set 5 TIME	Set 5 REPS	Set 6 TIME	Set 6 REPS
Plank Double Leg Lateral Hops						
Floor Pendulum Oblique Twists						
Jump Rope						
Floor Push-Up Plank						

Date:
Routine: Work-to-rest ratio: 60/20 sec.

Exercise	Set 1 TIME	Set 1 REPS	Set 2 TIME	Set 2 REPS	Set 3 TIME	Set 3 REPS
Floor Oblique Crunch						
Jump Rope						
Floor Push-Up Plank						
Burpees						

Exercise	Set 4 TIME	Set 4 REPS	Set 5 TIME	Set 5 REPS	Set 6 TIME	Set 6 REPS
Floor Oblique Crunch						
Jump Rope						
Floor Push-Up Plank						
Burpees						

Date:
Routine: Recovery Day

Upper and Lower Body

Block 1 — Upper Body

Date:

Routine: Upper Body
Work-to-rest ratio: 60/20 sec.
Active rest: Jump Rope 30 sec. between exercises 1 and 2

Exercise	Set 1 LBS	Set 1 REPS	Set 2 LBS	Set 2 REPS	Set 3 LBS	Set 3 REPS
Dumbbell Chest Press						
Triceps Dips						
Dumbbell Deltoid Lateral Raise						
Dumbbell Deltoid Frontal Raise						

Exercise	Set 4 LBS	Set 4 REPS	Set 5 LBS	Set 5 REPS	Set 6 LBS	Set 6 REPS
Dumbbell Chest Press						
Triceps Dips						
Dumbbell Deltoid Lateral Raise						
Dumbbell Deltoid Frontal Raise						

Block 2 — Lower Body

Date:

Routine: Lower Body
Work-to-rest ratio: 60/20 sec.
Active rest: Jumping Jacks 30 sec. between exercises 2 and 3

Exercise	Set 1 LBS	Set 1 REPS	Set 2 LBS	Set 2 REPS	Set 3 LBS	Set 3 REPS
Dumbbell Sumo Squat						
Dumbbell Back Lunges						
Dumbbell Calf Raises						
Side Lying Leg Raises						

Exercise	Set 4 LBS	Set 4 REPS	Set 5 LBS	Set 5 REPS	Set 6 LBS	Set 6 REPS
Dumbbell Sumo Squat						
Dumbbell Back Lunges						
Dumbbell Calf Raises						
Side Lying Leg Raises						

Block 3 — Full Body

Date:

Routine: Full Body
Work-to-rest ratio: 60/20 sec.
Active rest: High Knees 30 sec. between exercises 2 and 3

Exercise	Set 1 LBS	Set 1 REPS	Set 2 LBS	Set 2 REPS	Set 3 LBS	Set 3 REPS
Dumbbell Biceps Curl						
Triceps Dips						
Dumbbell Squat						
Dumbbell Back Lunges						

Exercise	Set 4 LBS	Set 4 REPS	Set 5 LBS	Set 5 REPS	Set 6 LBS	Set 6 REPS
Dumbbell Biceps Curl						
Triceps Dips						
Dumbbell Squat						
Dumbbell Back Lunges						

Block 4 — Split

Date:

Routine: Split
Time-under-tension: 20 reps in 60 sec.
Active rest: Jump Rope 30 sec. between exercises 1 and 2

Exercise	Set 1 LBS	Set 1 REPS	Set 2 LBS	Set 2 REPS	Set 3 LBS	Set 3 REPS
Dumbbell Back Rows						
Dumbbell Chest Press						
Dumbbell Back Diagonal Lunges						
Dumbbell Pilates Squat						

Exercise	Set 4 LBS	Set 4 REPS	Set 5 LBS	Set 5 REPS	Set 6 LBS	Set 6 REPS
Dumbbell Back Rows						
Dumbbell Chest Press						
Dumbbell Back Diagonal Lunges						
Dumbbell Pilates Squat						

Block 5 — Split

Date:

Routine: Split
Time-under-tension: 20 reps in 60 sec.
Active rest: Burpees 30 sec. between exercises 1 and 2

Exercise	Set 1 LBS	Set 1 REPS	Set 2 LBS	Set 2 REPS	Set 3 LBS	Set 3 REPS
Chin-Ups						
Dumbbell Triceps Kick Back						
Dumbbell Sumo Squat						
Butt Hip Raises						

Exercise	Set 4 LBS	Set 4 REPS	Set 5 LBS	Set 5 REPS	Set 6 LBS	Set 6 REPS
Chin-Ups						
Dumbbell Triceps Kick Back						
Dumbbell Sumo Squat						
Butt Hip Raises						

Block 6 — Recovery Day

Date:

Routine: Recovery Day

Compound and Functional

Routine 1

Date						
Routine	Work-to-rest ratio: 60/20 sec. Active rest: Burpees for 30 sec. between exercises 2 and 3					
Exercise	Set 1		Set 2		Set 3	
	TIME	REPS	TIME	REPS	TIME	REPS
TRX Atomic Push-Up						
TRX Suspended V Pike						
TRX Atomic Push-Up						
TRX Tornado Twist						
	Set 4		Set 5		Set 6	
	TIME	REPS	TIME	REPS	TIME	REPS
TRX Atomic Push-Up						
TRX Suspended V Pike						
TRX Atomic Push-Up						
TRX Tornado Twist						

Routine 2

Date						
Routine	Work-to-rest ratio: 60/20 sec. Active rest: Floor Bear Crawls for 30 sec. between exercises 1 and 2					
Exercise	Set 1		Set 2		Set 3	
	TIME	REPS	TIME	REPS	TIME	REPS
Explosive Start Throws						
BOSU Reverse Burpee and Roll-Up Squat Hop-Up						
TRX Hack Squat						
TRX Suspended Side Plank with Twist						
	Set 4		Set 5		Set 6	
	TIME	REPS	TIME	REPS	TIME	REPS
Explosive Start Throws						
BOSU Reverse Burpee and Roll-Up Squat Hop-Up						
TRX Hack Squat						
TRX Suspended Side Plank with Twist						

Routine 3

Date						
Routine	Work-to-rest ratio: 60/20 sec. Active rest: Jump Rope for 30 sec. between exercises 1 and 2					
Exercise	Set 1		Set 2		Set 3	
	TIME	REPS	TIME	REPS	TIME	REPS
BOSU Balance Trainer High Knees with One Leg On and One Leg Off						
TRX Suspended Side Plank with Twist and Pike						
Sideways Hurdle Running						
Powerdive Push-Up						
	Set 4		Set 5		Set 6	
	TIME	REPS	TIME	REPS	TIME	REPS
BOSU Balance Trainer High Knees with One Leg On and One Leg Off						
TRX Suspended Side Plank with Twist and Pike						
Sideways Hurdle Running						
Powerdive Push-Up						

Routine 4

Date						
Routine	Work-to-rest ratio: 60/20 sec. Active rest: Mountain Climbers for 30 sec. between exercises 2 and 3					
Exercise	Set 1		Set 2		Set 3	
	TIME	REPS	TIME	REPS	TIME	REPS
TRX Superman						
TRX Atomic Push-Up						
Tuck Jumps						
BOSU Forward Burpee with Squat Hop-Up Onto BOSU						
	Set 4		Set 5		Set 6	
	TIME	REPS	TIME	REPS	TIME	REPS
TRX Superman						
TRX Atomic Push-Up						
Tuck Jumps						
BOSU Forward Burpee with Squat Hop-Up Onto BOSU						

Routine 5

Date						
Routine	Work-to-rest ratio: 60/20 sec. Active rest: High Knees for 30 sec. between exercises 2 and 3					
Exercise	Set 1		Set 2		Set 3	
	TIME	REPS	TIME	REPS	TIME	REPS
Your Choice						
Your Choice						
Your Choice						
Your Choice						
	Set 4		Set 5		Set 6	
	TIME	REPS	TIME	REPS	TIME	REPS
Your Choice						
Your Choice						
Your Choice						
Your Choice						

Routine 6

Date						
Routine	Recovery Day					
Exercise	Set 1		Set 2		Set 3	
	TIME	REPS	TIME	REPS	TIME	REPS
	Set 4		Set 5		Set 6	
	TIME	REPS	TIME	REPS	TIME	REPS

Endurance

Mon	Tue	Wed	Thu	Fri	Sat	Sun
3-mile run	9×200	Rest or easy run	35 min. tempo	Rest or easy run	Rest	5k test race

Week 5

You now have four weeks of training under your belt—congratulations! From week five on out, perform six sets of each exercise with a brief rest in between. These final weeks of training push your endurance, which will pay off in spades on the obstacle course. Just as others are starting to tire, you'll be kicking it into the next gear.

The workout emphasis for this week is as follows: 50 percent muscular endurance, 30 percent power, 20 percent strength.

Cardio and Core

Date _____ Routine: Work-to-rest ratio: 60/10 sec.

Exercise	Set 1 TIME	Set 1 REPS	Set 2 TIME	Set 2 REPS	Set 3 TIME	Set 3 REPS
Mountain Climbers						
Floor V Crunch (Single Leg)						
Floor Reverse Crunch						
Power Jacks						

Exercise	Set 4 TIME	Set 4 REPS	Set 5 TIME	Set 5 REPS	Set 6 TIME	Set 6 REPS
Mountain Climbers						
Floor V Crunch (Single Leg)						
Floor Reverse Crunch						
Power Jacks						

Date _____ Routine: Work-to-rest ratio: 60/10 sec.

Exercise	Set 1 TIME	Set 1 REPS	Set 2 TIME	Set 2 REPS	Set 3 TIME	Set 3 REPS
Jumping Jacks						
Burpees						
Floor Oblique Crunch						
Floor Pendulum Oblique Twists						

Exercise	Set 4 TIME	Set 4 REPS	Set 5 TIME	Set 5 REPS	Set 6 TIME	Set 6 REPS
Jumping Jacks						
Burpees						
Floor Oblique Crunch						
Floor Pendulum Oblique Twists						

Date _____ Routine: Work-to-rest ratio: 60/10 sec.

Exercise	Set 1 TIME	Set 1 REPS	Set 2 TIME	Set 2 REPS	Set 3 TIME	Set 3 REPS
Lateral Jumping						
Floor Forward Crunch						
Stability Ball Forward Crunch						
Plank Lateral Jacks						

Exercise	Set 4 TIME	Set 4 REPS	Set 5 TIME	Set 5 REPS	Set 6 TIME	Set 6 REPS
Lateral Jumping						
Floor Forward Crunch						
Stability Ball Forward Crunch						
Plank Lateral Jacks						

Date _____ Routine: Work-to-rest ratio: 60/10 sec.

Exercise	Set 1 TIME	Set 1 REPS	Set 2 TIME	Set 2 REPS	Set 3 TIME	Set 3 REPS
High Knees in Place						
Burpees						
Floor V Crunch (Single Leg)						
Floor Push-Up Plank						

Exercise	Set 4 TIME	Set 4 REPS	Set 5 TIME	Set 5 REPS	Set 6 TIME	Set 6 REPS
High Knees in Place						
Burpees						
Floor V Crunch (Single Leg)						
Floor Push-Up Plank						

Date _____ Routine: Work-to-rest ratio: 60/10 sec.

Exercise	Set 1 TIME	Set 1 REPS	Set 2 TIME	Set 2 REPS	Set 3 TIME	Set 3 REPS
Mountain Climbers						
Floor Oblique Crunch						
Forward and Backward Jumping						
Jumping Jacks						

Exercise	Set 4 TIME	Set 4 REPS	Set 5 TIME	Set 5 REPS	Set 6 TIME	Set 6 REPS
Mountain Climbers						
Floor Oblique Crunch						
Forward and Backward Jumping						
Jumping Jacks						

Date _____ Routine: Recovery Day

Upper and Lower Body

Upper Body

Date:

Routine: Upper Body
Time-under-tension: 20 reps in 60 sec.
Active rest: Mountain Climbers 30 sec. between exercises 1 and 2

Exercise	Set 1 LBS	Set 1 REPS	Set 2 LBS	Set 2 REPS	Set 3 LBS	Set 3 REPS
Dumbbell Incline Chest Press						
Chin-Ups						
Dumbbell Shoulder Press						
Dumbbell Triceps Skull Crusher						

Exercise	Set 4 LBS	Set 4 REPS	Set 5 LBS	Set 5 REPS	Set 6 LBS	Set 6 REPS
Dumbbell Incline Chest Press						
Chin-Ups						
Dumbbell Shoulder Press						
Dumbbell Triceps Skull Crusher						

Lower Body

Date:

Routine: Lower Body
Time-under-tension: 20 reps in 60 sec.
Active rest: High Knees 30 sec. between exercises 1 and 2

Exercise	Set 1 LBS	Set 1 REPS	Set 2 LBS	Set 2 REPS	Set 3 LBS	Set 3 REPS
Dumbbell Calf Raises						
Dumbbell Squat						
Dumbbell Forward Lunges						
Dumbbell Pilates Squat						

Exercise	Set 4 LBS	Set 4 REPS	Set 5 LBS	Set 5 REPS	Set 6 LBS	Set 6 REPS
Dumbbell Calf Raises						
Dumbbell Squat						
Dumbbell Forward Lunges						
Dumbbell Pilates Squat						

Full Body

Date:

Routine: Full Body
Time-under-tension: 20 reps in 60 sec.
Active rest: Burpees 30 sec. between exercises 3 and 4

Exercise	Set 1 LBS	Set 1 REPS	Set 2 LBS	Set 2 REPS	Set 3 LBS	Set 3 REPS
Dumbbell Triceps Overhead Extension						
Dumbbell Incline Biceps Curl						
Dumbbell Squat						
Dumbbell Back Lunges						

Exercise	Set 4 LBS	Set 4 REPS	Set 5 LBS	Set 5 REPS	Set 6 LBS	Set 6 REPS
Dumbbell Triceps Overhead Extension						
Dumbbell Incline Biceps Curl						
Dumbbell Squat						
Dumbbell Back Lunges						

Split (Jump Rope)

Date:

Routine: Split
Work-to-rest ratio: 60/10 sec.
Active rest: Jump Rope 30 sec. between exercises 2 and 3

Exercise	Set 1 LBS	Set 1 REPS	Set 2 LBS	Set 2 REPS	Set 3 LBS	Set 3 REPS
Dumbbell Pilates Squat						
Pull-Ups						
Butt Hip Raises						
Dumbbell Back Rows						

Exercise	Set 4 LBS	Set 4 REPS	Set 5 LBS	Set 5 REPS	Set 6 LBS	Set 6 REPS
Dumbbell Pilates Squat						
Pull-Ups						
Butt Hip Raises						
Dumbbell Back Rows						

Split (High Knees)

Date:

Routine: Split
Work-to-rest ratio: 60/10 sec.
Active rest: High Knees 30 sec. between exercises 2 and 3

Exercise	Set 1 LBS	Set 1 REPS	Set 2 LBS	Set 2 REPS	Set 3 LBS	Set 3 REPS
Dumbbell Biceps Curl						
Dumbbell Sumo Squat						
Dumbbell Triceps Overhead Extension						
Dumbbell Back Lunges						

Exercise	Set 4 LBS	Set 4 REPS	Set 5 LBS	Set 5 REPS	Set 6 LBS	Set 6 REPS
Dumbbell Biceps Curl						
Dumbbell Sumo Squat						
Dumbbell Triceps Overhead Extension						
Dumbbell Back Lunges						

Recovery Day

Date:

Routine: Recovery Day

Compound and Functional

Date:

Routine: Work-to-rest ratio: 60/10 sec. Active rest: Burpees for 30 sec. between exercises 2 and 3

Exercise	Set 1		Set 2		Set 3	
	TIME	REPS	TIME	REPS	TIME	REPS
Lateral Jump to Box						
Squat Throws						
Circle Shoulder Raises						
Tuck Jumps						
	Set 4		Set 5		Set 6	
	TIME	REPS	TIME	REPS	TIME	REPS
Lateral Jump to Box						
Squat Throws						
Circle Shoulder Raises						
Tuck Jumps						

Date:

Routine: Work-to-rest ratio: 60/10 sec. Active rest: Jump Rope for 30 sec. between exercises 2 and 3

Exercise	Set 1		Set 2		Set 3	
	TIME	REPS	TIME	REPS	TIME	REPS
TRX Suspended V Pike						
TRX Hack Squat						
Floor Bear Crawls						
Kneeling to Standing Battling Ropes						
	Set 4		Set 5		Set 6	
	TIME	REPS	TIME	REPS	TIME	REPS
TRX Suspended V Pike						
TRX Hack Squat						
Floor Bear Crawls						
Kneeling to Standing Battling Ropes						

Date:

Routine: Work-to-rest ratio: 60/10 sec. Active rest: Jumping Jacks for 30 sec. between exercises 1 and 2

Exercise	Set 1		Set 2		Set 3	
	TIME	REPS	TIME	REPS	TIME	REPS
TRX Suspended Leg Circles						
TRX Suspended Walking Plank						
TRX Atomic Push-Up						
TRX Superman						
	Set 4		Set 5		Set 6	
	TIME	REPS	TIME	REPS	TIME	REPS
TRX Suspended Leg Circles						
TRX Suspended Walking Plank						
TRX Atomic Push-Up						
TRX Superman						

Date:

Routine: Work-to-rest ratio: 60/10 sec. Active rest: Burpees for 30 sec. between exercises 2 and 3

Exercise	Set 1		Set 2		Set 3	
	TIME	REPS	TIME	REPS	TIME	REPS
Lateral Hurdle Jumps						
BOSU Forward Burpee with Squat Hop-Up Onto BOSU						
Powerdive Push-Up						
TRX Seated Pull-Up						
	Set 4		Set 5		Set 6	
	TIME	REPS	TIME	REPS	TIME	REPS
Lateral Hurdle Jumps						
BOSU Forward Burpee with Squat Hop-Up Onto BOSU						
Powerdive Push-Up						
TRX Seated Pull-Up						

Date:

Routine: Work-to-rest ratio: 60/10 sec. Active rest: High Knees for 30 sec. between exercises 2 and 3

Exercise	Set 1		Set 2		Set 3	
	TIME	REPS	TIME	REPS	TIME	REPS
BOSU Balance Trainer High Knees with One Leg On and One Leg Off						
Forward Hurdle Running						
Lateral Jump to Box						
TRX Atomic Push-Up						
	Set 4		Set 5		Set 6	
	TIME	REPS	TIME	REPS	TIME	REPS
BOSU Balance Trainer High Knees with One Leg On and One Leg Off						
Forward Hurdle Running						
Lateral Jump to Box						
TRX Atomic Push-Up						

Date:

Routine: Recovery Day

Endurance

Mon	Tue	Wed	Thu	Fri	Sat	Sun
3-mile run	7×400	Rest or easy run	40 min. tempo	Rest	5-mile fast	75 min. run

Week 6

You might feel like you're in the best shape of your life as you begin week six. Don't slack off now. Continue performing six reps of each exercise; really push yourself on the active rest. The training outcomes for this week are distributed as follows: 50 percent strength, 30 percent power, 20 percent muscular endurance.

Cardio and Core

Date: ___   **Routine:** Work-to-rest ratio: 60/10 sec.

Exercise	Set 1 Time	Set 1 Reps	Set 2 Time	Set 2 Reps	Set 3 Time	Set 3 Reps
Floor Oblique Crunch						
TRX Side Elbow Plank						
Floor V Crunch (Single Leg)						
Burpees						

Exercise	Set 4 Time	Set 4 Reps	Set 5 Time	Set 5 Reps	Set 6 Time	Set 6 Reps
Floor Oblique Crunch						
TRX Side Elbow Plank						
Floor V Crunch (Single Leg)						
Burpees						

Date: ___   **Routine:** Work-to-rest ratio: 60/10 sec.

Exercise	Set 1 Time	Set 1 Reps	Set 2 Time	Set 2 Reps	Set 3 Time	Set 3 Reps
Jumping Jacks						
High Knees in Place						
Floor Reverse Crunch						
Forward and Backward Jumping						

Exercise	Set 4 Time	Set 4 Reps	Set 5 Time	Set 5 Reps	Set 6 Time	Set 6 Reps
Jumping Jacks						
High Knees in Place						
Floor Reverse Crunch						
Forward and Backward Jumping						

Date: ___   **Routine:** Work-to-rest ratio: 60/10 sec.

Exercise	Set 1 Time	Set 1 Reps	Set 2 Time	Set 2 Reps	Set 3 Time	Set 3 Reps
Floor Forward Crunch						
Plank Double Leg Lateral Hops						
Floor Pendulum Oblique Twists						
Floor Oblique Crunch						

Exercise	Set 4 Time	Set 4 Reps	Set 5 Time	Set 5 Reps	Set 6 Time	Set 6 Reps
Floor Forward Crunch						
Plank Double Leg Lateral Hops						
Floor Pendulum Oblique Twists						
Floor Oblique Crunch						

Date: ___   **Routine:** Work-to-rest ratio: 60/10 sec.

Exercise	Set 1 Time	Set 1 Reps	Set 2 Time	Set 2 Reps	Set 3 Time	Set 3 Reps
Burpees						
Jump Rope						
Stability Ball Forward Crunch						
Floor Oblique Crunch						

Exercise	Set 4 Time	Set 4 Reps	Set 5 Time	Set 5 Reps	Set 6 Time	Set 6 Reps
Burpees						
Jump Rope						
Stability Ball Forward Crunch						
Floor Oblique Crunch						

Date: ___   **Routine:** Work-to-rest ratio: 60/10 sec.

Exercise	Set 1 Time	Set 1 Reps	Set 2 Time	Set 2 Reps	Set 3 Time	Set 3 Reps
Plank Double Leg Lateral Hops						
Jumping Jacks						
Floor Push-Up Plank						
Floor Oblique Crunch						

Exercise	Set 4 Time	Set 4 Reps	Set 5 Time	Set 5 Reps	Set 6 Time	Set 6 Reps
Plank Double Leg Lateral Hops						
Jumping Jacks						
Floor Push-Up Plank						
Floor Oblique Crunch						

Date: ___   **Routine:** Recovery Day

Upper and Lower Body

Date:

Routine: Upper Body
Work-to-rest ratio: 60/10 sec.
Active rest: Jump Rope 30 sec. between exercises 1 and 2

Exercise	Set 1 LBS	Set 1 REPS	Set 2 LBS	Set 2 REPS	Set 3 LBS	Set 3 REPS
Triceps Dips						
Dumbbell Biceps Curl						
Chin-Ups						
Dumbbell Shoulder Press						

Exercise	Set 4 LBS	Set 4 REPS	Set 5 LBS	Set 5 REPS	Set 6 LBS	Set 6 REPS
Triceps Dips						
Dumbbell Biceps Curl						
Chin-Ups						
Dumbbell Shoulder Press						

Date:

Routine: Lower Body
Work-to-rest ratio: 60/10 sec.
Active rest: Jumping Jacks 30 sec. between exercises 2 and 3

Exercise	Set 1 LBS	Set 1 REPS	Set 2 LBS	Set 2 REPS	Set 3 LBS	Set 3 REPS
Dumbbell Sumo Squat						
Side Lying Leg Raises						
Dumbbell Calf Raises						
Dumbbell Back Diagonal Lunges						

Exercise	Set 4 LBS	Set 4 REPS	Set 5 LBS	Set 5 REPS	Set 6 LBS	Set 6 REPS
Dumbbell Sumo Squat						
Side Lying Leg Raises						
Dumbbell Calf Raises						
Dumbbell Back Diagonal Lunges						

Date:

Routine: Full Body
Work-to-rest ratio: 60/10 sec.
Active rest: High Knees 30 sec. between exercises 2 and 3

Exercise	Set 1 LBS	Set 1 REPS	Set 2 LBS	Set 2 REPS	Set 3 LBS	Set 3 REPS
Dumbbell Incline Chest Press						
Dumbbell Back Flies						
Dumbbell Squat						
Side Lying Leg Raises						

Exercise	Set 4 LBS	Set 4 REPS	Set 5 LBS	Set 5 REPS	Set 6 LBS	Set 6 REPS
Dumbbell Incline Chest Press						
Dumbbell Back Flies						
Dumbbell Squat						
Side Lying Leg Raises						

Date:

Routine: Split
Time-under-tension: 20 reps in 60 sec.
Active rest: Jumping Jacks 30 sec. between exercises 1 and 2

Exercise	Set 1 LBS	Set 1 REPS	Set 2 LBS	Set 2 REPS	Set 3 LBS	Set 3 REPS
Dumbbell Deltoid Lateral Raise						
Dumbbell Forward Lunges						
Dumbbell Triceps Kick Back						
Dumbbell Pilates Squat						

Exercise	Set 4 LBS	Set 4 REPS	Set 5 LBS	Set 5 REPS	Set 6 LBS	Set 6 REPS
Dumbbell Deltoid Lateral Raise						
Dumbbell Forward Lunges						
Dumbbell Triceps Kick Back						
Dumbbell Pilates Squat						

Date:

Routine: Split
Time-under-tension: 20 reps in 60 sec.
Active rest: Floor Bear Crawls 30 sec. between exercises 1 and 2

Exercise	Set 1 LBS	Set 1 REPS	Set 2 LBS	Set 2 REPS	Set 3 LBS	Set 3 REPS
Dumbbell Calf Raises						
Dumbbell Back Flies						
Chin-Ups						
Dumbbell Chest Press						

Exercise	Set 4 LBS	Set 4 REPS	Set 5 LBS	Set 5 REPS	Set 6 LBS	Set 6 REPS
Dumbbell Calf Raises						
Dumbbell Back Flies						
Chin-Ups						
Dumbbell Chest Press						

Date:

Routine: Recovery Day

Endurance

Mon	Tue	Wed	Thu	Fri	Sat	Sun
3-mile run	10×200	Rest or easy run	40 min. tempo	Rest	6-mile fast	85 min. run

Compound and Functional

Routine 1
Work-to-rest ratio: 55/20 sec.
Active rest: Burpees for 30 sec. between exercises 2 and 3

Exercise	Set 1 TIME	Set 1 REPS	Set 2 TIME	Set 2 REPS	Set 3 TIME	Set 3 REPS
Diagonal Forward Bounding						
TRX Hack Squat						
TRX Atomic Push-Up						
Sideways Hurdle Running						

Exercise	Set 4 TIME	Set 4 REPS	Set 5 TIME	Set 5 REPS	Set 6 TIME	Set 6 REPS
Diagonal Forward Bounding						
TRX Hack Squat						
TRX Atomic Push-Up						
Sideways Hurdle Running						

Routine 2
Work-to-rest ratio: 55/20 sec.
Active rest: Floor Bear Crawls for 30 sec. between exercises 1 and 2

Exercise	Set 1 TIME	Set 1 REPS	Set 2 TIME	Set 2 REPS	Set 3 TIME	Set 3 REPS
TRX Suspended Side Plank with Twist						
TRX Atomic Push-Up						
TRX Superman						
TRX Suspended Walking Plank						

Exercise	Set 4 TIME	Set 4 REPS	Set 5 TIME	Set 5 REPS	Set 6 TIME	Set 6 REPS
TRX Suspended Side Plank with Twist						
TRX Atomic Push-Up						
TRX Superman						
TRX Suspended Walking Plank						

Routine 3
Work-to-rest ratio: 55/20 sec.
Active rest: Jump Rope for 30 sec. between exercises 1 and 2

Exercise	Set 1 TIME	Set 1 REPS	Set 2 TIME	Set 2 REPS	Set 3 TIME	Set 3 REPS
TRX Suspended V Pike						
TRX Suspended Side Plank with Twist and Pike						
BOSU Reverse Burpee and Roll-Up Squat Hop-Up						
BOSU Balance Trainer High Knees with One Leg On and One Leg Off						

Exercise	Set 4 TIME	Set 4 REPS	Set 5 TIME	Set 5 REPS	Set 6 TIME	Set 6 REPS
TRX Suspended V Pike						
TRX Suspended Side Plank with Twist and Pike						
BOSU Reverse Burpee and Roll-Up Squat Hop-Up						
BOSU Balance Trainer High Knees with One Leg On and One Leg Off						

Routine 4
Work-to-rest ratio: 60/10 sec.
Active rest: Mountain Climbers for 30 sec. between exercises 2 and 3

Exercise	Set 1 TIME	Set 1 REPS	Set 2 TIME	Set 2 REPS	Set 3 TIME	Set 3 REPS
Lateral Jump to Box						
Forward Hurdle Running						
Circle Shoulder Raises						
Powerdive Push-Up						

Exercise	Set 4 TIME	Set 4 REPS	Set 5 TIME	Set 5 REPS	Set 6 TIME	Set 6 REPS
Lateral Jump to Box						
Forward Hurdle Running						
Circle Shoulder Raises						
Powerdive Push-Up						

Routine 5
Work-to-rest ratio: 60/10 sec.
Active rest: Jumping Jacks for 30 sec. between exercises 2 and 3

Exercise	Set 1 TIME	Set 1 REPS	Set 2 TIME	Set 2 REPS	Set 3 TIME	Set 3 REPS
Powerdive Push-Up						
Squat Throws						
TRX Tornado Twist						
BOSU Forward Burpee with Squat Hop-Up Onto BOSU						

Exercise	Set 4 TIME	Set 4 REPS	Set 5 TIME	Set 5 REPS	Set 6 TIME	Set 6 REPS
Powerdive Push-Up						
Squat Throws						
TRX Tornado Twist						
BOSU Forward Burpee with Squat Hop-Up Onto BOSU						

Routine 6
Recovery Day

Week 7

Two more weeks until race day. Time to get your *Grrr* on during weeks seven and eight!

The focus for training this week is 50 percent power, 30 percent muscular endurance, and 20 percent strength.

Cardio and Core

Block 1

Date						
Routine	Work-to-rest ratio: 60/5 sec.					

Exercise	Set 1 TIME	Set 1 REPS	Set 2 TIME	Set 2 REPS	Set 3 TIME	Set 3 REPS
Floor Side Elbow Plank						
Jumping Jacks						
Floor Oblique Crunch						
Power Jacks						

Exercise	Set 4 TIME	Set 4 REPS	Set 5 TIME	Set 5 REPS	Set 6 TIME	Set 6 REPS
Floor Side Elbow Plank						
Jumping Jacks						
Floor Oblique Crunch						
Power Jacks						

Block 2

Date						
Routine	Work-to-rest ratio: 60/5 sec.					

Exercise	Set 1 TIME	Set 1 REPS	Set 2 TIME	Set 2 REPS	Set 3 TIME	Set 3 REPS
Floor Forward Crunch						
Floor Reverse Crunch						
Floor Oblique Crunch						
Floor V Crunch (Single Leg)						

Exercise	Set 4 TIME	Set 4 REPS	Set 5 TIME	Set 5 REPS	Set 6 TIME	Set 6 REPS
Floor Forward Crunch						
Floor Reverse Crunch						
Floor Oblique Crunch						
Floor V Crunch (Single Leg)						

Block 3

Date						
Routine	Work-to-rest ratio: 60/5 sec.					

Exercise	Set 1 TIME	Set 1 REPS	Set 2 TIME	Set 2 REPS	Set 3 TIME	Set 3 REPS
Burpees						
Power Jacks						
Plank Double Leg Lateral Hops						
Forward and Backward Jumping						

Exercise	Set 4 TIME	Set 4 REPS	Set 5 TIME	Set 5 REPS	Set 6 TIME	Set 6 REPS
Burpees						
Power Jacks						
Plank Double Leg Lateral Hops						
Forward and Backward Jumping						

Block 4

Date						
Routine	Work-to-rest ratio: 60/5 sec.					

Exercise	Set 1 TIME	Set 1 REPS	Set 2 TIME	Set 2 REPS	Set 3 TIME	Set 3 REPS
Power Jacks						
Stability Ball Praying Mantis						
High Knees in Place						
Floor Forward Crunch						

Exercise	Set 4 TIME	Set 4 REPS	Set 5 TIME	Set 5 REPS	Set 6 TIME	Set 6 REPS
Power Jacks						
Stability Ball Praying Mantis						
High Knees in Place						
Floor Forward Crunch						

Block 5

Date						
Routine	Work-to-rest ratio: 60/5 sec.					

Exercise	Set 1 TIME	Set 1 REPS	Set 2 TIME	Set 2 REPS	Set 3 TIME	Set 3 REPS
Floor Oblique Crunch						
Floor Pendulum Oblique Twists						
Jump Rope						
Lateral Jumping						

Exercise	Set 4 TIME	Set 4 REPS	Set 5 TIME	Set 5 REPS	Set 6 TIME	Set 6 REPS
Floor Oblique Crunch						
Floor Pendulum Oblique Twists						
Jump Rope						
Lateral Jumping						

Block 6

Date						
Routine	Recovery Day					

Exercise	Set 1 TIME	Set 1 REPS	Set 2 TIME	Set 2 REPS	Set 3 TIME	Set 3 REPS

Exercise	Set 4 TIME	Set 4 REPS	Set 5 TIME	Set 5 REPS	Set 6 TIME	Set 6 REPS

Upper and Lower Body

Date							Date							Date						
Routine	Upper Body Time-under-tension: 30 reps in 60 sec. Active rest: Burpees 30 sec. between exercises 1 and 2						Routine	Lower Body Time-under-tension: 30 reps in 60 sec. Active rest: Jump Rope 30 sec. between exercises 1 and 2						Routine	Full Body Time-under-tension: 30 reps in 60 sec. Active rest: High Knees 30 sec. between exercises 3 and 4					
Exercise	Set 1		Set 2		Set 3		Exercise	Set 1		Set 2		Set 3		Exercise	Set 1		Set 2		Set 3	
	LBS	REPS	LBS	REPS	LBS	REPS		LBS	REPS	LBS	REPS	LBS	REPS		LBS	REPS	LBS	REPS	LBS	REPS
Dumbbell Incline Chest Press							Dumbbell Pilates Squat							Dumbbell Biceps Curl						
Dumbbell Shoulder Press							Dumbbell Sumo Squat							Dumbbell Calf Raises						
Chin-Ups							Dumbbell Back Lunges							Dumbbell Triceps Kick Back						
Triceps Dips							Dumbbell Forward Lunges							Dumbbell Back Diagonal Lunges						
	Set 4		Set 5		Set 6			Set 4		Set 5		Set 6			Set 4		Set 5		Set 6	
	LBS	REPS	LBS	REPS	LBS	REPS		LBS	REPS	LBS	REPS	LBS	REPS		LBS	REPS	LBS	REPS	LBS	REPS
Dumbbell Incline Chest Press							Dumbbell Pilates Squat							Dumbbell Biceps Curl						
Dumbbell Shoulder Press							Dumbbell Sumo Squat							Dumbbell Calf Raises						
Chin-Ups							Dumbbell Back Lunges							Dumbbell Triceps Kick Back						
Triceps Dips							Dumbbell Forward Lunges							Dumbbell Back Diagonal Lunges						

Date							Date							Date						
Routine	Split Work-to-rest ratio: 60/5 sec. Active rest: Jumping Jacks 30 sec. between exercises 2 and 3						Routine	Split Work-to-rest ratio: 60/5 sec. Active rest: Jumping Jacks 30 sec. between exercises 2 and 3						Routine	Recovery Day					
Exercise	Set 1		Set 2		Set 3		Exercise	Set 1		Set 2		Set 3		Exercise	Set 1		Set 2		Set 3	
	LBS	REPS	LBS	REPS	LBS	REPS		LBS	REPS	LBS	REPS	LBS	REPS		LBS	REPS	LBS	REPS	LBS	REPS
Pull-Ups							Your Choice													
Dumbbell Shoulder Press							Your Choice													
Dumbbell Squat							Your Choice													
Butt Hip Raises							Your Choice													
	Set 4		Set 5		Set 6			Set 4		Set 5		Set 6			Set 4		Set 5		Set 6	
	LBS	REPS	LBS	REPS	LBS	REPS		LBS	REPS	LBS	REPS	LBS	REPS		LBS	REPS	LBS	REPS	LBS	REPS
Pull-Ups							Your Choice													
Dumbbell Shoulder Press							Your Choice													
Dumbbell Squat							Your Choice													
Butt Hip Raises							Your Choice													

Compound and Functional

Date _____ Routine: Work-to-rest ratio: 60/5 sec. Active rest: Burpees for 30 sec. between exercises 2 and 3

Exercise	Set 1 TIME	Set 1 REPS	Set 2 TIME	Set 2 REPS	Set 3 TIME	Set 3 REPS
Lateral Box Push-Offs						
Tuck Jumps						
TRX Superman						
Powerdive Push-Up						

Exercise	Set 4 TIME	Set 4 REPS	Set 5 TIME	Set 5 REPS	Set 6 TIME	Set 6 REPS
Lateral Box Push-Offs						
Tuck Jumps						
TRX Superman						
Powerdive Push-Up						

Date _____ Routine: Work-to-rest ratio: 60/5 sec. Active rest: Jump Rope for 30 sec. between exercises 2 and 3

Exercise	Set 1 TIME	Set 1 REPS	Set 2 TIME	Set 2 REPS	Set 3 TIME	Set 3 REPS
TRX Suspended Side Plank with Twist and Pike						
TRX Hack Squat						
TRX Atomic Push-Up						
BOSU Forward Burpee with Squat Hop-Up Onto BOSU						

Exercise	Set 4 TIME	Set 4 REPS	Set 5 TIME	Set 5 REPS	Set 6 TIME	Set 6 REPS
TRX Suspended Side Plank with Twist and Pike						
TRX Hack Squat						
TRX Atomic Push-Up						
BOSU Forward Burpee with Squat Hop-Up Onto BOSU						

Date _____ Routine: Work-to-rest ratio: 60/5 sec. Active rest: Jumping Jacks for 30 sec. between exercises 1 and 2

Exercise	Set 1 TIME	Set 1 REPS	Set 2 TIME	Set 2 REPS	Set 3 TIME	Set 3 REPS
Floor Bear Crawls						
Explosive Start Throws						
Lateral Jump to Box						
Lateral Hurdle Jumps						

Exercise	Set 4 TIME	Set 4 REPS	Set 5 TIME	Set 5 REPS	Set 6 TIME	Set 6 REPS
Floor Bear Crawls						
Explosive Start Throws						
Lateral Jump to Box						
Lateral Hurdle Jumps						

Date _____ Routine: Work-to-rest ratio: 60/5 sec. Active rest: Burpees for 30 sec. between exercises 2 and 3

Exercise	Set 1 TIME	Set 1 REPS	Set 2 TIME	Set 2 REPS	Set 3 TIME	Set 3 REPS
Circle Shoulder Raises						
TRX Tornado Twist						
TRX Suspended V Pike						
TRX Suspended Side Plank with Twist						

Exercise	Set 4 TIME	Set 4 REPS	Set 5 TIME	Set 5 REPS	Set 6 TIME	Set 6 REPS
Circle Shoulder Raises						
TRX Tornado Twist						
TRX Suspended V Pike						
TRX Suspended Side Plank with Twist						

Date _____ Routine: Work-to-rest ratio: 60/5 sec. Active rest: Jump Rope for 30 sec. between exercises 2 and 3

Exercise	Set 1 TIME	Set 1 REPS	Set 2 TIME	Set 2 REPS	Set 3 TIME	Set 3 REPS
TRX Hack Squat						
TRX Atomic Push-Up						
TRX Tornado Twist						
TRX Superman						

Exercise	Set 4 TIME	Set 4 REPS	Set 5 TIME	Set 5 REPS	Set 6 TIME	Set 6 REPS
TRX Hack Squat						
TRX Atomic Push-Up						
TRX Tornado Twist						
TRX Superman						

Date _____ Routine: Recovery Day

Endurance

Mon	Tue	Wed	Thu	Fri	Sat	Sun
3-mile run	8×400	Rest or easy run	45 min. tempo	Rest	6-mile fast	90 min. run

Week 8

Race day is right around the corner. During week eight, continue attacking your workouts as if you're out on the course. As you perform each exercise, visualize yourself going through a similar obstacle that requires similar movements. For instance, if you're doing planks, imagine yourself crawling under barbed wire. If you're doing chin-ups, visualize yourself scaling a high wall.

Cardio and Core

Date							Date							Date						
Routine	Work-to-rest ratio: 60/5 sec.						Routine	Work-to-rest ratio: 60/5 sec.						Routine	Work-to-rest ratio: 60/5 sec.					
Exercise	Set 1		Set 2		Set 3		Exercise	Set 1		Set 2		Set 3		Exercise	Set 1		Set 2		Set 3	
	TIME	REPS	TIME	REPS	TIME	REPS		TIME	REPS	TIME	REPS	TIME	REPS		TIME	REPS	TIME	REPS	TIME	REPS
Stability Ball Praying Mantis							Lateral Jumping							Floor Reverse Crunch						
Floor Oblique Crunch							Forward and Backward Jumping							Mountain Climbers						
Floor Pendulum Oblique Twists							High Knees in Place							Floor Push-Up Plank						
Floor Reverse Crunch							Burpees							Forward and Backward Jumping						
	Set 4		Set 5		Set 6			Set 4		Set 5		Set 6			Set 4		Set 5		Set 6	
	TIME	REPS	TIME	REPS	TIME	REPS		TIME	REPS	TIME	REPS	TIME	REPS		TIME	REPS	TIME	REPS	TIME	REPS
Stability Ball Praying Mantis							Lateral Jumping							Floor Reverse Crunch						
Floor Oblique Crunch							Forward and Backward Jumping							Mountain Climbers						
Floor Pendulum Oblique Twists							High Knees in Place							Floor Push-Up Plank						
Floor Reverse Crunch							Burpees							Forward and Backward Jumping						

Date							Date							Date						
Routine	Work-to-rest ratio: 60/5 sec.						Routine	Work-to-rest ratio: 60/5 sec.						Routine	Recovery Day					
Exercise	Set 1		Set 2		Set 3		Exercise	Set 1		Set 2		Set 3		Exercise	Set 1		Set 2		Set 3	
	TIME	REPS	TIME	REPS	TIME	REPS		TIME	REPS	TIME	REPS	TIME	REPS		TIME	REPS	TIME	REPS	TIME	REPS
Jump Rope							Floor Reverse Crunch													
Floor Reverse Crunch							Mountain Climbers													
Plank Double Leg Lateral Hops							Floor Push-Up Plank													
Floor Reverse Crunch							Plank Double Leg Lateral Hops													
	Set 4		Set 5		Set 6			Set 4		Set 5		Set 6			Set 4		Set 5		Set 6	
	TIME	REPS	TIME	REPS	TIME	REPS		TIME	REPS	TIME	REPS	TIME	REPS		TIME	REPS	TIME	REPS	TIME	REPS
Jump Rope							Floor Reverse Crunch													
Floor Reverse Crunch							Mountain Climbers													
Plank Double Leg Lateral Hops							Floor Push-Up Plank													
Floor Reverse Crunch							Plank Double Leg Lateral Hops													

Upper and Lower Body

Date							Date							Date						
Routine	Upper Body Work-to-rest ratio: 60/5 sec. Active rest: High Knees 30 sec. between exercises 1 and 2						Routine	Lower Body Work-to-rest ratio: 60/5 sec. Active rest: Mountain Climbers 30 sec. between exercises 2 and 3						Routine	Full Body Work-to-rest ratio: 60/5. Active rest: Burpees 30 sec. between exercises 2 and 3					
Exercise	Set 1		Set 2		Set 3		Exercise	Set 1		Set 2		Set 3		Exercise	Set 1		Set 2		Set 3	
	LBS	REPS	LBS	REPS	LBS	REPS		LBS	REPS	LBS	REPS	LBS	REPS		LBS	REPS	LBS	REPS	LBS	REPS
Dumbbell Triceps Overhead Extension							Dumbbell Squat							Dumbbell Back Rows						
Chin-Ups							Dumbbell Back Lunges							Dumbbell Chest Flies						
Dumbbell Chest Press							Side Lying Leg Raises							Dumbbell Sumo Squat						
Dumbbell Biceps Curl							Dumbbell Calf Raises							Dumbbell Forward Lunges						
	Set 4		Set 5		Set 6			Set 4		Set 5		Set 6			Set 4		Set 5		Set 6	
	LBS	REPS	LBS	REPS	LBS	REPS		LBS	REPS	LBS	REPS	LBS	REPS		LBS	REPS	LBS	REPS	LBS	REPS
Dumbbell Triceps Overhead Extension							Dumbbell Squat							Dumbbell Back Rows						
Chin-Ups							Dumbbell Back Lunges							Dumbbell Chest Flies						
Dumbbell Chest Press							Side Lying Leg Raises							Dumbbell Sumo Squat						
Dumbbell Biceps Curl							Dumbbell Calf Raises							Dumbbell Forward Lunges						

Date							Date							Date						
Routine	Split Time-under-tension: 30 reps in 60 sec. Active rest: Jump Rope 30 sec. between exercises 1 and 2						Routine	Split Time-under-tension: 30 reps in 60 sec. Active rest: Burpees 30 sec. between exercises 1 and 2						Routine	Recovery Day					
Exercise	Set 1		Set 2		Set 3		Exercise	Set 1		Set 2		Set 3		Exercise	Set 1		Set 2		Set 3	
	LBS	REPS	LBS	REPS	LBS	REPS		LBS	REPS	LBS	REPS	LBS	REPS		LBS	REPS	LBS	REPS	LBS	REPS
Dumbbell Shoulder Press							Dumbbell Triceps Skull Crusher													
Dumbbell Pilates Squat							Dumbbell Pilates Squat													
Dumbbell Deltoid Lateral Raise							Dumbbell Incline Biceps Curl													
Butt Hip Raises							Dumbbell Calf Raises													
	Set 4		Set 5		Set 6			Set 4		Set 5		Set 6			Set 4		Set 5		Set 6	
	LBS	REPS	LBS	REPS	LBS	REPS		LBS	REPS	LBS	REPS	LBS	REPS		LBS	REPS	LBS	REPS	LBS	REPS
Dumbbell Shoulder Press							Dumbbell Triceps Skull Crusher													
Dumbbell Pilates Squat							Dumbbell Pilates Squat													
Dumbbell Deltoid Lateral Raise							Dumbbell Incline Biceps Curl													
Butt Hip Raises							Dumbbell Calf Raises													

Endurance

Mon	Tue	Wed	Thu	Fri	Sat	Sun
2-mile run	6×200	30 min. tempo	Rest or easy run	Rest	Rest	5k race

Compound and Functional

Routine 1

Date: _____

Routine: Work-to-rest ratio: 60/5 sec. Active rest: Burpees for 30 sec. between exercises 2 and 3

Exercise	Set 1 TIME	Set 1 REPS	Set 2 TIME	Set 2 REPS	Set 3 TIME	Set 3 REPS
TRX Atomic Push-Up						
TRX Hack Squat						
Circle Shoulder Raises						
TRX Seated Pull-Up						

Exercise	Set 4 TIME	Set 4 REPS	Set 5 TIME	Set 5 REPS	Set 6 TIME	Set 6 REPS
TRX Atomic Push-Up						
TRX Hack Squat						
Circle Shoulder Raises						
TRX Seated Pull-Up						

Routine 2

Date: _____

Routine: Work-to-rest ratio: 60/5 sec. Active rest: Floor Bear Crawls for 30 sec. between exercises 1 and 2

Exercise	Set 1 TIME	Set 1 REPS	Set 2 TIME	Set 2 REPS	Set 3 TIME	Set 3 REPS
Squat Throws						
TRX Suspended Side Plank with Twist						
Diagonal Forward Bounding						
BOSU Balance Trainer High Knees with One Leg On and One Leg Off						

Exercise	Set 4 TIME	Set 4 REPS	Set 5 TIME	Set 5 REPS	Set 6 TIME	Set 6 REPS
Squat Throws						
TRX Suspended Side Plank with Twist						
Diagonal Forward Bounding						
BOSU Balance Trainer High Knees with One Leg On and One Leg Off						

Routine 3

Date: _____

Routine: Work-to-rest ratio: 60/5 sec. Active rest: High Knees for 30 sec. between exercises 1 and 2

Exercise	Set 1 TIME	Set 1 REPS	Set 2 TIME	Set 2 REPS	Set 3 TIME	Set 3 REPS
Lateral Box Push-Offs						
TRX Suspended Walking Plank						
TRX Seated Pull-Up						
BOSU Reverse Burpee and Roll-Up Squat Hop-Up						

Exercise	Set 4 TIME	Set 4 REPS	Set 5 TIME	Set 5 REPS	Set 6 TIME	Set 6 REPS
Lateral Box Push-Offs						
TRX Suspended Walking Plank						
TRX Seated Pull-Up						
BOSU Reverse Burpee and Roll-Up Squat Hop-Up						

Routine 4

Date: _____

Routine: Work-to-rest ratio: 60/5 sec. Active rest: Mountain Climbers for 30 sec. between exercises 2 and 3

Exercise	Set 1 TIME	Set 1 REPS	Set 2 TIME	Set 2 REPS	Set 3 TIME	Set 3 REPS
TRX Superman						
BOSU Forward Burpee with Squat Hop-Up Onto BOSU						
Powerdive Push-Up						
Floor Bear Crawls						

Exercise	Set 4 TIME	Set 4 REPS	Set 5 TIME	Set 5 REPS	Set 6 TIME	Set 6 REPS
TRX Superman						
BOSU Forward Burpee with Squat Hop-Up Onto BOSU						
Powerdive Push-Up						
Floor Bear Crawls						

Routine 5

Date: _____

Routine: Work-to-rest ratio: 60/5 sec. Active rest: Mountain Climbers for 30 sec. between exercises 2 and 3

Exercise	Set 1 TIME	Set 1 REPS	Set 2 TIME	Set 2 REPS	Set 3 TIME	Set 3 REPS
Circle Shoulder Raises						
Floor Bear Crawls						
BOSU Reverse Burpee and Roll-Up Squat Hop-Up						
TRX Seated Pull-Up						

Exercise	Set 4 TIME	Set 4 REPS	Set 5 TIME	Set 5 REPS	Set 6 TIME	Set 6 REPS
Circle Shoulder Raises						
Floor Bear Crawls						
BOSU Reverse Burpee and Roll-Up Squat Hop-Up						
TRX Seated Pull-Up						

Routine 6

Date: _____

Routine: Recovery Day

Index